P9-DNA-165

The press weighs in on Edward Jackowski's fitness programs:

"Whether you take a fitness class or work out at home using exercises from books or videos, chances are your plan isn't targeted for you. And because of that, it may not be toning your problem areas quickly enough—or worse, it may be bulking up the very parts you'd like to slim . . . Now there's [Jackowski's] breakthrough approach to toning based on your body's natural shape." —*Redbook*

"An effective and practical plan to get you in the best shape of your life." —*Men's Journal*

"It's easy to exercise right with Edward's way, and if you do, you'll slim down and tone up in far less time." —*Prevention*

"Want to reshape your shape? Knowing your body type may make all the difference. . . . Jackowski has built a business out of assessing body types." —*Vogue*

"Edward is an innovator in the industry. [He] takes bodies that fairly jiggle with flab and turns them into the kind of bodies people don't dare kick sand at—at the beach or anyplace else." —*Newsday*

"What's this? You've been exercising like a maniac only to find that your thighs are thicker and your butt bigger? . . . You may be doing exercises that build muscle in your problem areas faster than they help you burn fat. Jackowski strikes back with a system of fitness formulas based on body types." —*Bridal Guide*

"[Ed Jackowski] claims his trademarked fitness regimen based on body types is 'the only program in existence designed to help a person improve his shape.' Normally we'd dismiss such egotism, but the truth is the program works (we've tried it)—and it is unique." —*Playboy*

"[Jackowski] could make even the most reluctant exerciser a believer." —*W*

"[Jackowski's] the guy who fitness journalists call for exercise and workout advice because this guy knows his stuff. He knows the body inside and out. He speaks physiology and translates it into terms anyone can understand. He's the teacher you wished you had in school, and when it comes to aerobic and anaerobic conditioning and jumping rope, believe me, this guy is the master." —*Fit*

"Your health club won't tell you this, but the trendy machine you're working out on might not make you fit and could even injure you if you don't use it right. By the way, did you notice your butt's getting bigger? As gyms are realizing that results are the single best motivation, they're starting to mimic themes similar to Edward Jackowski's." —*New York*

Escape Your Shape: How to Work Out Smarter, Not Harder

EDWARD J. JACKOWSKI, Ph.D.,
author of *Hold It! You're Exercising Wrong*

Illustrations by Youzell Jeffers

A FIRESIDE BOOK
Published by Simon & Schuster
NEW YORK LONDON TORONTO SYDNEY SINGAPORE

This publication contains the opinions and ideas of its author. It is intended to provide helpful and informative material on the subjects addressed in the publication. The reader should consult his or her medical, health or other competent professional before adopting any of the suggestions in this book or drawing inferences from it.

The author and publisher specifically disclaim all responsibility for any liability, loss or risk, personal or otherwise, which is incurred as a consequence, directly or indirectly, of the use and application of any of the contents of this book.

FIRESIDE
Rockefeller Center
1230 Avenue of the Americas
New York, NY 10020

Copyright © 2001 by Edward J. Jackowski, Ph.D.
All rights reserved,
including the right of reproduction
in whole or in part in any form.

Fireside and colophon are registered trademarks
of Simon & Schuster, Inc.

Designed by Elina D. Nudelman

Manufactured in the United States of America

9   10   8

Library of Congress Cataloging-in-Publication Data

Jackowski, Edward.
Escape your shape : how to work out smarter, not harder /
Edward J. Jackowski.
p.   cm.
Includes index.
1. Reducing exercises.   2. Somatotypes.   I. Title.
RA781.6.J33 2001
613.7'1—dc21   2001020309

ISBN 0-7432-1144-8

Acknowledgments

My greatest thanks go to my staff at Exude Fitness in New York City, especially Jason and Lee Ross, for their dedication to getting our clients fit and allowing me the time necessary to write this book. I also want to thank Lara Ross and my brother Thomas, whose patience, insight and organizational skills helped me to see things in a different light, one that you the reader can better relate to and understand.

To my clients, who had the smarts to listen and follow my guidance over the years, and who can now proudly and definitely say, "I escaped my shape." Special thanks to the entire staff at Simon & Schuster, especially my editor, Lisa Considine, whose confidence and respect for me as a business professional and writer made writing this book so enjoyable. And to my agent, Gareth Esersky, at the Carol Mann Agency, who was able to influence the powers that be that this book was very much needed for anyone looking to improve the way he or she looks and feels.

Contents

## PART I

HOW TO WORK OUT SMARTER, NOT HARDER

For years, health clubs, fitness equipment man-
ufacturers and all of the so-called fitness ex-
perts have been inventing new ways to
mentally and physically stimulate us while we
exercise. Granted, many of them do succeed in
motivating people to exercise—at least initially.
You can plug headphones into treadmills, elliptical trainers and StairMasters and tune into
your favorite shows. You can take yoga and Pi-
lates classes, learn how to kick-box and even
belly dance. We go to extremes in search of motivation.

For the past twenty years I have focused on
one thing and one thing only: motivating people to exercise by improving the way their body
looks, feels and functions through exercise. Two
decades have shown me that great results are

the best motivators around. How do I get results? Through a revolutionary system that guides my clients to the best exercise for their body type. It is no secret that we are not all built the same, so how could we all possibly exercise the same way and expect to look great? We can't. One size does not fit all. No one exercise program works for everyone. That is what *Escape Your Shape* is all about.

Say you and three total strangers are sitting in a doctor's office complaining of skin irritations, and the doctor sized up the three of you with a look and made his pronouncement: "Since you all have some skin irritation on your arm, just take this prescription and it should go away. Thanks for coming in." What would you think? More important, would you take this doctor's advice? I wouldn't. But, curiously, we accept and follow the advice of people who tell us to take spinning classes when our legs are disproportionately large to begin with. Or we lift heavy weights to combat osteoporosis and as a result bulk our arms until they are too big for our bodies. There is an alternative. There is a way to trim down problem areas, to strengthen and tone without bulking to achieve your specific fitness goals.

Everyone wants to improve his or her body. Most people are willing to do practically anything in order to "look" better—crash diets, fat-burning pills, fat-blocking pills, liquid diets, protein diets, no-fat diets, working out for two to three hours a day, fasting and even undergoing surgery in the form of liposuction. They will use whatever means necessary to reach their goals.

You would think that with all of the magazines, books and television shows touting exercise, fitness and healthy lifestyles, we would be a somewhat fit and healthy nation. The reality is that although we are more aware of the benefits of regular exercise, few have a clue how to exercise *properly*—and as a result never meet their goals. We all want to look and feel our best, exercise regularly, eat properly and exude confidence in both our personal and professional lives, but though many try, very few achieve. This book will help you reach these goals. I am the messenger, and although sometimes you may not like what I tell you, if you listen, I promise you will escape your shape. If you follow my guidance, you will begin to see your body change for the better within 30 days.

Let me tell you a story about a woman who came to me for help. Susan, a typical Spoon body type, has a tendency to put on weight and mass in the lower part of her body. She naturally wants to reduce the size of those problem areas. To kick things off I ask Susan about her current exercise routine and she tells me she takes step classes and spinning classes and with her "trainer" does lunges, squats and leg presses with lots of weights. I ask her how long she has been working out this way, and she tells me five years.

"Susan," I ask, "have your legs and lower body gotten any smaller over this time?"

"No," Susan is quick to respond. "Actually my jeans are tighter than when I started and I just don't understand. Why haven't I lost any mass or size with all this exercise? I know I'm eating right."

"Susan," I said, "you are a Spoon and the exercises you are performing are not ones I recommend for you because you have a tendency to add muscle mass faster than you burn fat, especially in your lower body." Susan then explains her trainer's rationale: the more muscle she builds, the more fat she burns. That much is true, but what her trainer failed to mention was than in order to burn more fat and raise her metabolic rate significantly, she needed to increase her muscle mass by at least 20 percent! Nor did he tell her that no one can convert fat into muscle, biologically speaking. The fat that lies on the inner and outer parts of legs, the hips and the rear end can never be turned to muscle or "firmed" since fat and muscle are different substances; fat doesn't turn to muscle and muscle does not turn to fat.

"Tell me, Susan, did your 'trainer' ever show you before-and-after photos of clients with bodies like yours before you started working with him? Did you speak to any of his clients who told you they were thrilled with the results of his program?"

He had not, of course. What Susan and many others fail to recognize is that there is a big difference between a trainer who can demonstrate the proper form for a particular exercise and someone who can train you to change your body for the better. To convince Susan further I ask her if she thought weight lifting could bulk you. Remarkably, Susan says she doesn't know. "Susan," I ask, "if you took a marathon runner's workout and a body builder's workout and switched them, would their bodies remain the same?"

"No," Susan says, a realization dawning on her.

"So do weights bulk you?"

"I guess so," Susan says. Based on her original theory—that weights do not bulk you—you could become a competitive body builder by swimming, jogging or playing badminton. Obviously, it doesn't work that way. Still, Susan does not want to give up her step or spinning classes. I tell her that's okay but explain that sticking to them means that she'll never have the body she desires.

"What do you mean?" Susan moans.

"Susan, *I'm* not telling you that you're exercising wrong. Your body is. I'm just the messenger. Don't complain about the *size* of your legs, hips and rear end, because until you start exercising correctly for your body type, you will never, ever change your body to your level of satisfaction." How do I know this? I know this because it would have worked already! She has been exercising this way for the past five years without the results she wants.

It took twenty minutes to convince Susan that she needed to start exercising according to her body type. And it was worth it. It's not easy to break a five-year habit. Today, Susan is slimmer down below and one of my favorite graduates. Everywhere she goes, she talks endlessly about Exude Fitness (www.exude.com).

Susan is just like thousands of exercisers out there. The reason why Susan did not want to give up her step classes is that she did not know what else to do. Still others are attached to their current workout because they're confident they can do it or are simply scared to try something new. After they follow my program, their attitudes undergo a remarkable change.

My goal is to get you to look and feel better in a short period of time because the most effective way to build and sustain motivation in *any* individual is to show results—and fast! At that point, you will be self-motivated to continue.

Maybe you are not like Susan. Maybe you have not exercised for years. Maybe you think your body cannot change because you're genetically programmed to have big arms or big legs. You are wrong. You may be genetically programmed to put fat and mass on certain parts of your body, but you have complete control to choose the *way* you exercise. And you can choose to exercise right for your body type. This book is not about possessing a perfect body; it is about getting your body to look its best. It's about finally getting results for your hard work. Anyone, despite body shape, age or weight, can dramatically improve their body by exercising according to body type.

I want to instill that in order to escape your shape, you are going to need a plan. Not a plan that works for a week, month or year, but a foolproof exercise plan that works for the rest of your life. The plan is as important as the actual exercise program that you will perform. This plan involves taking the necessary steps to ensure that you stick with your program. You cannot jump ahead, skip around and attempt to do it "your way." We all want the end result, but there're no two ways about it, it takes hard work to get there. You can't skip from A to Z. I meet plenty of people who try to go from A to F, skip to M, maybe go to T and then skip to Z! Part of the reason they have trouble getting to Z is that they don't know what Z feels like. They've never been there! But you can get there with my plan. I am going to remind you throughout this book to stick to the plan; it is your personal roadmap for success. What I have realized over the past twenty years as a motivational coach and what I want to teach you is that the actual work involved in escaping your shape is not difficult. The only time that I have not seen a person's body change entirely to their satisfaction is when they don't stick to the plan, instead doing it their way.

Being fit is about getting up in the morning and embracing the day, feeling good about yourself and your life. My goal is to have you playing golf or tennis, gardening, hiking, biking and doing whatever else you want to do—effortlessly! When you are fit and feeling good about yourself, you can partake in your favorite activities for the love of the sport, not as a substitute for exercise. You will fight off stress, combat disease and depression and improve your immune system function. You'll also be more confident and attract positive people in your personal as well as professional lives. More important, you are going to have the strength to combat the curve balls that life will invariably throw at you.

I have written this book to share my years of experience with you so that you too can escape your shape. This book is written for all of you seeking to improve the way you look and feel, whether you are frustrated from exercising for years without seeing results or are exercising for the first time. I will personally walk you through every step, educating and motivating you along the way. I will share with you anecdotes and real stories of people like you, people like Susan. You will escape your shape and will look at exercise from an entirely different perspective.

## CHAPTER 1

What Does It Mean to Escape Your Shape?

I want you to imagine yourself in a room, an exercise room. You have an hour to perform a full-body exercise routine. That is, you have an hour to perform both aerobic and anaerobic exercise, improve your cardiovascular efficiency and strengthen your upper body, midsection and lower body. You'll also need to work on increasing your flexibility and range of motion and build endurance throughout your entire body. Your workout should include a warm-up, stretching, the right mix of aerobic and anaerobic exercise and a cooldown at the end. Did I also mention that I want you to exercise in such a fashion that improves the way your body looks, trimming your problem areas?

In this exercise room you have access to every piece of fitness equipment imaginable: steppers, treadmills, bikes, free weights, Cybex units, Nautilus stations, StairMasters, elliptical machines, and anything else you can think of. Are you ready? I am going to start the clock now, and remember you have only an hour.

Most folks, after freaking for a minute or two, start scrambling and thinking, What should I do first? My point is that virtually no one would do it correctly. Guess what? You cannot escape your shape or dramatically improve your fitness level unless you know what to do in that room.

Sure, some people would do certain exercises correctly or would know how to use some of the equipment, but very few people know how to assemble a complete workout using the tools supplied. My point is that if you don't know what to do, it doesn't matter what equipment you have access to. You may improve your cardiovascular health and strengthen some muscle groups, but you will fall way short of your goal if you're trying to transform your entire body or achieve full-body fitness.

Most people don't understand even the basics about fitness. Some, for instance, believe they're getting a complete workout by walking or running. Others think they're doing the same thing with free weights or yoga. Of course they're all forms of exercise, but in order to work out efficiently and effectively, maximizing the benefits to your health, your exercise program must improve and or maintain the five components of fitness: cardiovascular health, muscle strength, muscle endurance, flexibility and lean muscle to fat ratio. If your body type allows it, it's fine to run for your cardiovascular health, or lift weights to build strength, but you need to address the other components as well, each time you exercise.

Some operate under the misconception that golf, tennis, skiing and other sports are synonymous with fitness. I'm not saying you should stop doing the things you enjoy, since the fitter you are, the more you'll enjoy those activities. My point is that tennis, skiing and the like aren't exercise per se; they're activities. And though you may play tennis three times a week, you'll never achieve true fitness by only playing tennis. You won't improve your overall fitness by being more active. But you can be more active by becoming more fit.

In fact, one of the best ways to motivate yourself to exercise regularly is to train specifically to enhance your sports performance. With sport-specific training you can:

- reduce your risk of injury
- play at a more competitive level and derive more satisfaction from your improved performance

- enjoy the sport for its own sake, rather than relying on it for exercise
- extend the number of years you can play your favorite sport
- develop confidence in your physical abilities, and perhaps try other, more demanding activities

Aside from the physical, emotional, psychological and spiritual benefits of exercise, it's guaranteed to improve the way your body looks. You may even have a visual image of the way you want your body to appear when you look in the mirror completely naked. Do you look in the mirror now and say, "Ugh! Look at the size of my legs compared to my upper body!" Or, "Look at how my stomach sticks out!" It is essential that your exercise routine improves the way you look. Otherwise, why do it? What I've learned in my 20 years of work in the world of fitness is that everyone's body is different and everyone has different goals. If you want to improve your body and achieve a better-proportioned, toned, sleek body, you'll need an exercise program designed for your particular goals.

When you can enter that exercise room and work out under the conditions that I just laid out, you are on your way to escaping your shape! It is also important that you can perform your workout routine wherever that room happens to be. What do you do now when you are traveling and find yourself without access to a gym? If you can't get to your health club and are forced to exercise at home, will your workout be just as effective and efficient? How about if you miss the exercise class you wanted to take because you had to work late? Do you still work out, or do you blow it off because you really do not know how to exercise unless you are in that environment? In order to truly escape your shape, you *must* have a clear understanding of how to implement and modify your exercise plan so that you can do it anywhere and anytime!

You may be asking yourself why this is so important. The answer is, Because the most essential element needed to increase your fitness level and improve your body is *consistency!* If you cannot be regular with your fitness routine, it does not matter how effective your regimen may be; you will never escape your shape. That consistency is directly related to your fitness education. You need to learn how to properly exercise when you have only a half-hour rather than a full hour, and how to exercise when you have injured your arm, leg, foot or back. That's right, you can still get an effective workout despite whatever injury ails you. Without this fitness education, you may find yourself out of your usual environment or with an achy knee or back and have no idea of what to do.

If you've always been a runner and suddenly running isn't a fitness option because you have an achy back, for example, you may think there is nothing you can do. The reality of the situation is that there is a lot you can do. You may be able to alleviate your back pain and still run since it is more than likely the problem is that you do not stretch or do any abdominal exercises, which strengthen your back. A fitness education can solve this problem. When you are properly armed and understand how to work out in any circumstance, you have eliminated the possibility of failure. Consistency, coupled with a surefire workout routine based on your body type, yields success. Success today, next week, next month, next year, and for the rest of your life!

EVOLUTION OF THE BODY TYPES

I was fortunate to have parents who took the time to teach me all sports at a very young age. That coupled with my six siblings and a mother who would not allow any of us inside until it was dark paved the way for a very active life. I am a product of my environment. By the time I went to high school, I already possessed the skills and education to make exercise a part of my life. Most important, I always knew how to fit exercise into my schedule, despite any constraint that challenged me. I played football, golf, baseball, lacrosse, and basketball, ran track and snow- and water-skied. I was also one of the few athletes who trained regularly. Since I had size (I was naturally big-boned and very muscular), I stayed away from heavy weights and fo-cused my training on speed and endurance-type exercises such as skipping rope; doing sit-ups, chin-ups and push-ups and stretching. I soon started to develop training programs for each sport, using minimal fitness equipment and making sure that no matter where I traveled, I could always fit in my workouts. At 18 I started training other athletes and developing fitness programs for both my friends and fellow teammates. For a small fee I would work out with them and then design a fitness program for them to follow on their own.

I supported myself through business college working at a small fitness-equipment retail store. At the same time, I was tak-ing a class called entrepreneurial management. I needed to write a mock business plan and was getting a little desperate for an idea. One day, while working in the store, a big, burly gentle-man walked in and, right in front of my boss, asked me to demonstrate how to use a Universal multi-station weight ma-chine, which cost around $3,000. My boss's eyes lit up and I'm sure he expected me to get excited, too. If I made the sale, I'd have a 10 percent commission coming to me. I asked the cus-tomer why he wanted the machine and he said he was an avid tennis player and wanted to build his shoulders and upper body. I told him flat out that if he wanted to improve his tennis game that he was better off buying a jump rope and a simple dip unit to strengthen his shoulders. For about $100 he could achieve better results than he could with the $3,000 machine. "Besides," I said, "you're plenty big enough. What you need is endurance and foot speed and to trim down." I then offered to personally deliver the dip machine and show him how to stretch and use it properly. On my way home that evening, a lightbulb went off in my head, and Exude was born. My plan was to start a company that delivered fitness equipment, taught customers how to use it properly and then set them free. The next day in business class I asked an almost total stranger, this kid named Peter, for $400 to start a company and get incorporated. I promised him 20 percent of the company, but, thank God, he refused. Instead, he loaned me the money. Well, the rest is history, and that $400 launched one of the largest one-on-one motivational fitness companies in America. Thank you, Peter, wherever you are.

Years ago I began telling my clients, "That exercise is not most appropriate for your body type; this one is much better for you." It all started years before I ever classified or named the 4 types. It was intuitive for me. I would say things like, "Because you're top heavy, you should be doing this exercise to trim down in that area." It made sense. When they followed my advice, their bodies became better proportioned. In the beginning, to drum up business, I visited various health clubs and approached perfect strangers whose bodies looked out of proportion. I gave my business card to anyone who was bottom heavy or had a bulging stomach or whose legs were twigs compared to their massive upper bodies. I explained what I could do for them, and some of these people called and made appointments to come see me. During my initial meeting and evaluation, I would analyze the way they exercised. Aside from the fact that no one warmed up, then stretched, or cooled down after their workout, I was struck by two common problems. First off, none of the people who had poor flexibility *ever* stretched and they all had back pain. Second and most disturbing, there were an enormous number of men and women who exercised wrong for their bodies and got bigger in places they were trying to slim down. I saw highly motivated businesswomen who were built like body builders. They complained about how big they were and how they loathed the size of their arms, hips and thighs. In short, all of them were putting in the effort and exercising regularly, but they had little if anything to show for literally years of hard work. It never occurred to them that other exercises might help them achieve their goals. The number of clients with this problem was too great to ignore.

I decided to go to the library and do some research. I wanted to see why certain exercises built muscle and mass while others slimmed our bodies. In a nutshell, my research confirmed that aerobic activities, such as running, biking, swimming, jumping rope and rowing help to take mass off the body and that anaerobic exercise, things like weight lifting, sit-ups, calisthenics and push-ups help tone our muscles and add mass. The more resistance, tension or weights you use, the bigger your muscles get. I also discovered when you don't exercise a muscle, it simply shrinks. It does not turn to fat, as many people believe. Also, contrary to popular belief, muscle does **not** weigh more than fat. It's common sense: 100 pounds of fat, feathers, muscle, gold and potatoes all weigh the same! However, muscle is denser. That is, the space or volume that a pound of fat takes up in our bodies is nearly two to three times that of a pound of muscle.

It's no accident that marathon runners, swimmers and rowers are very lean. Nor is it coincidence that body builders, sprinters and speed skaters are very muscular and considerably larger. So, any logical person can deduct that the kind of exercise we engage in directly affects the way our body is shaped. We are not all built the same. Some of us have a tendency to bulk at certain regions of our body more readily than others. In order to change your body and ultimately look better proportioned the key is to match the exercise *and* the degree of resistance to your body type. Both are needed to affect positive change. For instance, if you are built like a Spoon (bottom heavy), you might choose biking for the aerobic component of your fitness routine. That's fine, but if you bike with high resistance or tension, you will actually increase the size of your legs because your body type has a tendency to add muscle faster than it can burn fat in that region of your body. The resistance component is just as important as your choice of exercise. If you do not believe me, take a look at most spinning instructors at your gym. Do you see small quadriceps muscles? I don't think so!

As my business grew, magazine editors and television producers began calling me for interviews. Initially I remember many a beauty or fitness editor objecting to my philosophy. They'd bristle, saying, "Edward, I'm not going to write that step classes or stair climbers will actually *increase* the size of some people's legs. Our magazine just ran a piece on how to have perfect legs or buns and everyone says that's the way to do it." Talking my talk wasn't enough to convince them, so I started lobbying members of the media who were doing those types of exercises and who looked like puffed-up bodybuilders to try it my way. I offered them a thirty-day program at no charge. We agreed that if I could change their body within thirty days, they would consider writing a piece in their magazine about their experience with Exude. Well, they *all* saw results and soon piece after piece ran in one fashion magazine after another. Suddenly they started to say things like "Maybe this guy Jackowski does know what he's talking about." It was success of a kind, but I knew that if I wanted to universalize my body-type system, I needed more credibility and exposure. I started writing fitness and lifestyle columns for any publication I could and self-published a booklet on what exercisers were doing wrong. It caught the eye of an editor at Simon & Schuster who asked me if I could expand it into a book. I wanted to get people's attention and help them stop and think before they went out there and flailed aimlessly with their workouts. I called it, *Hold It! You're Exercising Wrong.*

It unveiled my body-type methodology, outlining characteristics of each type and providing the dos and don'ts all in a single chapter. I took my experience in the industry and my years of observations, and concluded that people fell into one of 4 basic types: Hourglass, Spoon, Ruler or Cone. In addition, a handful of people, because they are overweight, are combinations of body types.

It was the first time that anyone in or outside of the fitness industry ever identified the different body builds. From that original classification grew the first and only body-type system to provide effective and individualized fitness regimens that improve the way your body looks—for both men and women.

However, I merely introduced my body-type methodology back then. Today, I have perfected exercise routines for each body type down to the smallest detail. This book is about what you need to do in order to improve your body, no matter how you are built. Have you ever noticed that most people who work out at your local gym or friends who announce that they have started a diet or exercise program really don't look any better than before? With this book in hand, you can be the exception.

Nevertheless, when it's finally said and done, the main reason we may be exercising wrong correlates with a lack of knowledge. That's the point of this book, to show you how to save time and energy and get you to the point where you follow a fitness prescription based upon your unique body type so that you'll like what you see when you look in the mirror.

IS THIS EXERCISE PROGRAM FOR ME?

Over the years, I have helped clients of all ages. I've coached people who suffer from eating disorders, obesity, diabetes, osteoporosis, herniated and slipped disks, knee replacements, hip replacements, heart conditions and high blood pressure. I've exercised with special population groups such as those with multiple sclerosis, muscular dystrophy, spinal injuries, and Down's syndrome. I have also worked with both professional and amateur athletes, people who loathe exercise, busy executives who travel constantly, children with attention deficit disorder and seniors who don't think that they can even get out of their beds. Every one of them dramatically improved their condition, increased their range of motion and improved their ability to perform their daily functions.

Many people who have an injury or medical condition are fearful of starting an exercise program because they think they "can't" work out without putting undue stress on their bodies. I can understand this dilemma, but I personally have never encountered *anyone* who was not physically capable of improving his or her fitness level despite his or her current condition. The reality of the situation is that many of these folks are unmotivated to begin with and use their injury as an excuse not to exercise. You have to possess the desire to get better, to do your homework, and to seek out people with the expertise you need in order to help get moving again.

I am always fascinated and gravely disappointed when I go to the beach and observe how little people move around. Oh sure, there is an occasional Frisbee toss going on, but in general, no one moves off the chair or blanket—until I arrive on the scene. I bring a volleyball net, paddles and footballs and I get everyone moving. However, I cannot be at every beach every day around the world. If I could I would! However, what I can do is supply you with the motivation and knowledge to get you self-motivated. Once you start moving and exercising properly and your body starts to take a turn for the better, you will become more active. Becoming and staying fit and active takes focus and determination. I am not unlike most of you. I have to watch what I eat and exercise regularly in order to look and feel great. I am just fortunate to know how to exercise in an effective and efficient manner. But I work at it, and you'll have to work consistently to make proper exercise a permanent part of your life.

Occasionally a new client comes to me with very modest expectations. He or she might say something like, "I just want to lose a little weight and size and feel better. I don't care that much if my legs or arms are trim. I'm fifty years old and married and I don't need to have that at this point of my life." My answer is always, "You'll lose weight, improve your health, feel better and improve your body at the same time. They're all the result of proper exercise. I can't give you one without the others." In other words, whether you are exercising for general health or to completely reshape your body, the program I have in mind for you is the same. You still have to warm up, stretch, do the correct amount and type of aerobic and anaerobic exercises based on your body type during your workload and then cool down afterward. There are certain rules and protocol that anyone who exercises must follow according to the American College of Sports Medicine (ACSM), the country's leading educational and research organization on the effects of exercise. Every fitness program I (or my staff at Exude) prescribe follows these guidelines. What is unique is how we warm up our clients, teach them to stretch and work them out. It is not dumb luck that in 20 years of business, there has never been a health claim against Exude. We must be doing something right!

In conclusion, I want you to know that this book and my program *is* for everyone. The magic of it is that it works for anyone who is willing to listen and apply its universal principles, whether you want to lose weight, tone up, increase your fitness level, get rid of a protruding stomach or flabby arms, trim your hips or thighs or even improve your posture. No matter what your current state of physical level is or your medical or orthopedic constraints are, you too can escape your shape!

## CHAPTER 2

Identifying Your Body Type

Everyone naturally has a body type or shape—Hourglass, Spoon, Ruler or Cone. These shapes are for the most part genetically predetermined. Recognizing and understanding your shape is the key to a successful fitness program. To achieve a leaner, more toned and better proportioned body you must recognize what you were born with and adjust your exercise plan accordingly. In my previous book, I articulated as no one had ever done before the difference between a standard cookie-cutter exercise program and a targeted exercise regime that would yield the desired results.

Here is an example of why understanding your body type *before* you begin exercising is critical to escaping your shape. It also explains why most people who are currently exercising fail to meet their goals. Say your wife playfully tweaks your ever-growing love handles or you find you no longer fit into your favorite jeans. What is your first reaction? If you are like the majority of Americans, you hit the gym and shell out good money for the advice of a personal trainer who looks like a clone of Arnold Schwarzenegger. He leads you through a series of exercises as he explains in a vague way what his particular exercises will do for you. You vow to attack the newest wave of steppers and lift weights for 2 hours every day. Simultaneously, you declare that nothing will pass through your lips save a carrot stick and tofu until the weight is lost. The experience of throwing yourself headlong into an exhausting physical and mental realignment *without a clear sense of the results you have a right to expect* leads, understandably, to failure. What's missing? Since you have decided that fitness will be a priority in your life, you need an exercise program that will deliver *results!* The first step in achieving these results is to recognize and identify your unique body type. The next step is to create an individualized plan that you will enjoy and master.

WHAT'S MY TYPE?

If you took a hard look at thousands of people's bodies, you'd notice the same thing I have: that people fall generally into 4 categories. Some people are bottom heavy, some are top heavy, some are naturally well proportioned and curvaceous and others have few curves. You too are either a Spoon, a Cone, an Hourglass or a Ruler. Whatever your body type is, it is basically determined by genetics. As you enter adulthood there are certain factors that influence how your body looks: how active or inactive you were growing up and are currently, the sports you participated in, your childhood and adolescent diet, how much time you spend sitting, and, most important, the variety of exercises you have performed over the years that have either enhanced or bulked certain regions of your body.

Your body type has nothing to do with how tall, short, skinny or fat you are. It has nothing to do with how much you weigh. Nor does it have anything to do with your innate athleticism, age, agility, coordination or fitness level. In fact, even your diet (food intake) has nothing to do with your body type. For example, if you are a Spoon and you are 5 foot 6 inches and weigh 140 pounds, you can diet and lose 10 or 15 pounds. But you won't significantly improve the way your body looks, especially your problem areas, by dieting alone. The only way I can transform you from a ladle to a demitasse spoon is by getting you to exercise properly for your type. You can be a fat Ruler, a thin Spoon or a skinny Hourglass, for example. No matter what your type, weight or fitness level, you can improve them.

Identifying your body type is simply a matter of observing how your weight is distributed on your frame. No one body type is better or worse than another. While you cannot change from one body type to another, you can improve your shape and make the best of your body type through proper exercise. Some of you may want to lose weight and inches throughout your body; others, just inches. Some will want to trim their thighs, stomach or other specific areas. Whatever your goals, it's paramount to identify your shape in order to exercise appropriately.

How to Identify Your Shape

First use the following questions to determine what your body type is. Then take a look at the illustrations of the four types. Do you recognize yourself? If you're still unsure, read the detailed profiles for each body type.

Do you tend to carry weight in both your upper and lower body, yet are more slender through the waist? Is there a significant difference between the circumference of your chest and your waist (or between your hips and waist)? Does your body appear balanced and curvaceous when you look in the mirror?

If so, you are an **HOURGLASS.**

Do you carry most of your weight in your hips, thighs and buttocks? Are you more slender on the top? Do you tend to gain weight or carry extra weight from the hips down? Do your eyes go directly to the lower half of your body when you look in the mirror?

If so, you are a **SPOON.**

Are you pretty much built straight up and down with very few curves? Is there little difference in the circumferences of your chest, waist and hips? Do you tend to put on weight around your midsection?

If so, you are a **RULER.**

Do you tend to carry most of your weight in your back, chest, arms and stomach? Are you more slender from the hips down?

If so, you are a **CONE.**

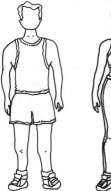
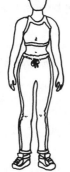

Hourglass

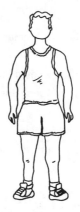
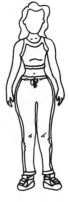

Spoon

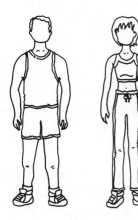

Ruler

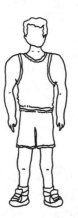
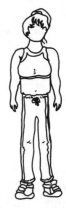

Cone

Important Facts and Tips

- Most women are either Spoons or Hourglasses.
- Most men are Rulers or Cones.
- If you are overweight, it may be more difficult to determine your actual body type. You may be caught between body types.
- You can be thin or fat for your body type, as well as short or tall for your body type.
- Although it is not very common, some women are flat-chested Hourglasses. Remember that determining your body type is about proportion. It is the total circumference of your back and chest that is relevant, not the size of your breasts.
- Some female Rulers naturally have big breasts, though it is not the norm.
- Although Spoon women are relatively small to medium chested, you could be a busty Spoon, though your hips and thighs will be comparatively larger.
- Your "diet" has very little to do with your body type, but it does directly influence your scale weight.

BODY-TYPE PERCENTAGES BY GENDER

Body Type	Female	Male
Hourglass	40%	20%
Spoon	30%	10%
Cone	10%	30%
Ruler	20%	40%

Still Not Sure?

If you are having problems determining your body type, it is probably because you are carrying extra weight. Fear not, simply follow the Hourglass workout until you shed off some of that weight. As you become slimmer and your natural shape begins to emerge, you can start adding some resistance and weight to your exercises. I find that many women look in the mirror and have eyes only for their problem areas. I can't tell you how many women misdiagnose their body type as a Spoon. They are all obsessed with the size of their thighs. A woman who is 5'8" and 170 pounds, who bulks in the arms and the thighs and is more slender around her stomach may *think* she is a Spoon because she has very big thighs. But in reality, she is an Hourglass with a tendency to bulk down below a little faster than she does up above. I call this type of woman a bottom-heavy Hourglass. She bulks both above and below but more on her bottom half. Because she is overweight by at least 20 pounds, a lot of that extra weight is emphasized below. She only thinks she is a Spoon because she dislikes that part of her body so much.

In truth, you're only temporarily caught between types. Deep down you are a pure Hourglass, Spoon, Ruler or Cone and you're overweight. You cannot be anything else. For example, you can't be a top-heavy Ruler, because someone who bulks only on top by definition is a Cone. Nor can you be a top-heavy Spoon, because that would make you an Hourglass. If you are larger throughout any one part of your body, you are either overweight and/or bulkier due to the type of exercises you have been performing.

TAKING MEASUREMENTS

I strongly recommend you take measurements prior to starting your body-type fitness routine. (See the section below for directions.) If possible, have a friend or colleague take them for you because it is very difficult to precisely or accurately measure yourself. Each time you turn and twist to get a measurement, it throws off the reading. Your measurements are important because they're a definitive indication of your body type. They are also a good way to track your progress so you can make adjustments to your workouts as necessary. You may find that quantifiable improvements come in inches, but not scale weight. If you are overweight, and need to lose *both* inches and weight, you may need to adjust your caloric intake and/or diet. Once you see your problem areas start to shrink, you will become even more motivated to continue with your workouts. I suggest that you record your measurements every 30 days.

Keeping track of your measurements will help you adjust your workouts to meet your goals. Let's say you are an Hourglass and two months into your workouts you notice that while you're losing inches from your hips and thighs, your upper arms and back aren't responding as well. That typically means that you are not doing enough of your upper-body routine and/or aerobic exercise. Knowing that, you can adjust your workouts so that your upper body begins to change at a faster pace. You may also find that after losing a certain number of inches throughout your body that you don't need to lose as much weight as you first thought. You may have started out thinking you needed to lose at least 15 pounds, but after two months find you have dropped two dress sizes though lost only 5 pounds. I have seen countless clients, both men and women, lose just a few pounds but more than 10 inches from their body.

How and Where to Take Your Measurements

Hand a friend a tape measure and record the circumference of the following*:

CHEST. Place the tape measure across the middle of your breasts or chest and around the circumference of your back; exhale before the measurement is recorded.

---

* Please note: Measure only on one side for upper thigh, knee, calf and arms. Make sure you measure the same side when measuring in the future.

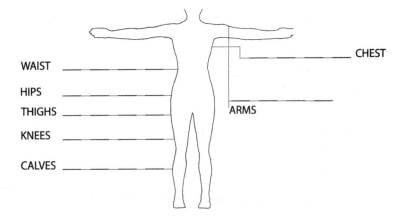

WAIST. Place the tape measure around your midsection, 1 inch above your belly button.

HIPS. Place the tape measure just below your hips, at the widest spot but still above your buttocks.

THIGHS. Measure the circumference of your upper thigh at the widest point, just barely under your buttocks.

KNEES. Measure 1 inch above the top of your kneecap.

CALVES. Measure in the middle of the calf, at the widest point.

ARMS. Measure on the upper arm just under the armpit, at the widest part.

Guidelines to Help Determine Your Body Type

1. HOURGLASSES will find that there is at *least* a 6-inch difference between their chest and waist and between their hips and waist. The girths of their chest and hips are within a couple of inches of one another. Common Hourglass measurements for chest, waist and hips respectively are 33-26-33, 36-30-38, 34-28-35, 39-32-38, or 42-35-44.

2. SPOONS will find that there is not a significant difference between the girths of their chest and waist but a significant difference between the girths of their hips and chest. For example, 34-30-38, 36-30-44, or 32-28-39.

3. RULERS will find that their chest, waist and hips are relatively close in measurement. Rulers are similar to Hourglasses but are less curvy and not as slender through the waist. For example, 34-30-35, 36-33-37, or 40-36-42.

4. Lastly, **CONES** will find that their chest and waist are relatively close in measurement and that their hips and thighs are significantly *smaller* than their chest. For example, 36-32-30, 40-36-33, or 34-30-29.

Remember, if you're overweight, you could be "caught" between body types. If you are, please follow the Hourglass workout until you trim down and your true body type is revealed.

THE HOURGLASS PROFILE

As an Hourglass, you will notice that you tend to put on weight or mass in both your upper and lower bodies while staying more slender through the waist. This applies whether you are a female or male. Generally, Hourglasses are trying to lose weight, mass or inches from both their upper and lower bodies. My Hourglass clients typically want to slim, tone and streamline their legs and the back of their arms (triceps). A lot of Hourglass women incorrectly label themselves Spoons. They either focus excessively on the size of their hips or thighs or are bottom-heavy Hourglasses. In other words, they bulk in both their upper and lower bodies, but do faster on the lower half. Hourglasses have to be especially careful with the type and amount of resistance exercise they perform with their lower and upper bodies.

One advantage of being an Hourglass is that you tend to lose and gain weight and mass evenly. Though it goes on fast, you can lose it quickly, too. Hourglasses can and should carry more scale weight than any other body type because your weight is distributed pretty evenly throughout your entire body. That's why a gal who is 5'6", large framed and well toned can look slender even at 150 pounds. Believe it or not, she'll look only about 135 *if* she exercises appropriately for an Hourglass. This is a classic case of someone who needs to lose inches rather than weight, a feat that cannot be achieved by dieting alone. In fact, losing inches, especially off your problem areas, can only be accomplished through proper exercise. So if you are a large-framed person, don't despair. True, you'll never be willowy, but you can be slender and fit and wear a size 8 with room to spare. As I tell many men and women who fall into this category, don't worry about your weight. The scale doesn't show inch loss, so you could be losing significant mass while the scale shows no improvement. Don't get depressed; for encouragement, rely on your shrinking waist and hips.

Let's look at an Hourglass named Melissa, who happens to be 40. She carries her 160 pounds on her 5'7" frame well, but could afford to lose 10 pounds. She thinks she should weigh 140 pounds, but she is very muscular and busty and her measurements prior to exercising for her body type were 38-32-40. She could easily shrink to 37-30-37, but years of exercising improperly have bulked her up. My assessment is that 150 pounds is a good weight for her. She will be able to maintain that weight easily without having to starve herself and, more important, maintain an exercise program in spite of her hectic lifestyle.

The trouble with Melissa's original weight-loss goal is that she hasn't weighed 140 since she was 19 years old, and she was a lot more active then. Today, it's unrealistic to think she can work out more than 4 days per week. She needs to separate reality from fantasy. The reality of the situation is that given her lifestyle, she has a limited amount of time to devote to exercise. To achieve her original target weight, she would have to exercise 6 days per week, go on a strict diet, quit going out with her business clients at night and stop eating and drinking out 5 days per week. That's just not going to happen. Sometimes what we want and what we are really able to do consistently don't match up. You need to be honest with yourself and make the best of your situation. At 150 pounds, Melissa will look better and healthier, improve her self-image and exude energy. At 140 pounds, she will be miserable, deprived and focusing on her weight rather than on being fit and healthy.

Problem Areas and Characteristics

Hourglasses are fortunate because they typically have strong bones and good muscle tone and are less susceptible to osteoporosis than other body types. As a group, senior Hourglasses have fewer fractures resulting from falls; they are built for high-contact and impact sports that require power, strength and speed. Also, sports or movements that require both upper- and lower-body strength are easier for Hourglasses than other body types. For very slim Hourglasses, jogging or running can be enjoyable, but for most, it is uncomfortable. They also tend to have good (sometimes excellent) flexibility throughout their entire body and generally do not have back problems because their abdominals are naturally strong. They have tapered legs and small ankles, though their calves may be muscular. Their problem areas tend to be the backs of the upper arms, the inner and outer thighs and the saddlebag region (just below the hips on the outside of the upper thigh). Some Hourglasses tend to put on weight around the lower portion of their abdominal region, which tends to add to their hip measurement. Most Hourglasses bulk and put on weight easily in both upper and lower regions and must be very careful not to add weights or resistance to their workouts.

If you're an Hourglass who's trying to slim down, hold off on adding weight or resistance to your exercise routine until you lose weight and mass. Even then you may notice you're bulking up more than you'd like. If so, cut back. Hourglasses almost always weigh considerably more than people think because of the way their weight is distributed on their frames.

Best Exercises for Escaping Your Hourglass Shape*

Jumping rope with a speed or peg rope

Stationary biking with light to moderate resistance and high RPMs (90 to 120)

Fast walking with little to no incline

Jogging or running for distance slowly (5 to 6 MPH without resistance or hills)

Ski machine at high speed with little to moderate tension for both upper and lower bodies

Elliptical machines with *no* resistance (only if you're not overweight)

Jumping jacks

Standing knee to opposite chest, L-kicks, leg-outs, one-legged leg lifts, and vertical scissors

Cybex, Nautilus or other weight machines with light weights and high reps

Upper-body routine with a 4-pound aerobic bar, doing push-outs, behind-the-neck presses, front presses, upright-rows, bicep curls, and tricep kickbacks

Dead lifts with little or no weight

Angled squats (if you're not overweight)

Leg extensions and leg curls with light weight and high reps

Swimming for distance (crawl stroke only)

---

* PLEASE NOTE: THE PRECEDING EXERCISES ARE RECOMMENDED FOR HOURGLASSES. REMEMBER THAT *NO ONE* EXERCISE CAN BRING TRUE FITNESS. YOU NEED TO PERFORM A FULL-BODY EXERCISE ROUTINE EACH AND EVERY TIME YOU WORK OUT. MAKE SURE THAT YOUR FITNESS REGIMEN IS MADE UP OF THE EXERCISES LISTED ABOVE. (SEE CHAPTER 7 FOR HOURGLASS WORKOUT ROUTINES AND INSTRUCTIONS ON HOW TO BEST PERFORM THE SUGGESTED EXERCISES.)

Exercises to Avoid if You Want
to Escape Your Hourglass Shape

Step classes

Spinning

High-impact aerobic or exercise classes

Kick-boxing

Squats, lunges, and leg presses

Inner-outer leg machines with high resistance

Stationary biking with high resistance

Walking, jogging or running on an incline, especially with hand weights
simultaneously

Ski machine with high resistance for both upper and lower bodies

Versa climbers

Jumping rope with a weighted rope

Stepper/stair climbers with resistance

All exercises using ankle weights

All lower-body exercises using high resistance or weights

All upper-body exercises using high resistance or weights

Roller blading on hills

Rowing with high resistance

Summary

As an Hourglass, your mantra is high reps, low resistance and low weights for both upper and lower bodies. High reps mean at least 25 to 50 repetitions for *each* of your exercises. As you slim down and lose weight and mass, you can increase resistance and weight. But you still *must* maintain your high reps for each exercise. Hourglasses who bulk very easily may have to keep the resistance and weights at a low level forever. If you currently engage in any of the above exercises and you're not willing to cut them out entirely, try to cut down on the number of times you perform them during the week. As you trim down, you can ease back into them.

THE SPOON PROFILE

Spoons tend to put on weight or mass in their hips and thighs and behind the knees. Those who are very overweight may even carry extra weight in their calves and ankles. Their upper bodies are not necessarily small, but considerably smaller than their lower bodies. Typically, if a Spoon is not overweight, the lower part of the leg, from the knee down is her best asset. Although it is rare, there are some male Spoons. Another distinctive feature of Spoons is that, unlike Hourglasses, they look heavier than their actual scale weight. Because most of their weight is concentrated in their lower half, others' eyes focus and fix primarily on this part of their bodies. It is important to note that as a Spoon, you bulk the fastest of all the body types from the hips down, so it's vital that each and every time you exercise you do so with absolutely *no* resistance or weights. I have seen thousands of women increase the size of their hips and thighs considerably by performing the wrong type of exercises. It's a horrible thought, but it's possible to bulk up from a size 10 to a 14 with the wrong exercises! A typical Spoon's measurements are 34-30-42. As I often tell Spoon women I work with, my goal is to take you from a ladle to a teaspoon. Your measurements should be 34-29-36. And you can do it! By exercising right for your body type. I have also found that generally sedentary Spoons who sit a lot can increase the size of their hips and thighs simply with the pressure and weight that they put on that region of the body. If they're not overweight, Spoons usually have very nice upper bodies and great upper abdominal muscles.

Problem Areas and Characteristics

Spoons typically have sleek upper bodies and have the best-looking arms of any of the body types. But because their upper bodies are considerably weaker and smaller in girth than other body types they're at greater risk for osteoporosis there, too. The flip side is that most Spoons, because of their muscle mass and weight below, are less likely to develop osteoporosis in their hips and lower limbs. Spoons typically have excellent lower flexibility and are good with sports or movements that require lower-body strength and coordination. Ballet dancers, tap dancers, and ballroom dancers are good examples of in-shape Spoons. They also typically shy away from sports that require upper-body strength because of their weaker upper bodies. If not vastly overweight, Spoons make good joggers, but unfortunately, jogging will not alter their bodies for the better. Nevertheless, it's a wonderful way for Spoons to lose and maintain weight loss.

Spoons usually have shortish legs and a long torso, thus making their legs appear larger than they actually are. If they lack good hamstring (back-of-the-legs) flexibility, they have a propensity for lower back pain. Overall, though, most Spoons do have great hamstring flexibility because of a higher fat content in that region. Their good flexibility means Spoons can work out vigorously with little risk of injury. They tend to carry the most mass on the saddlebag region (just below the hips and on the outside of the thigh), and some carry a lot of weight or mass in their hips. The good news for Spoons is that it is relatively easy to reduce these problem areas. Because of the disparity between their lower and upper bodies, once they start to slim down, the change for the better is hard to miss. The *key* is to perform a lot of light-resistance aerobic exercise combined with loads of lower-body calisthenics. With time and perseverance, Spoons can completely alter their shape for the better, but most likely will forever need to stay away from lower-body exercises with any resistance or weights.

Best Exercises for Escaping Your Spoon Shape*

Jumping rope with a speed rope
Stationary biking with light resistance only and high RPMs (90 to 120)

Jumping jacks

Ski machines with light resistance for lower body and high resistance for
upper body

Standing knee to opposite chest, L-kicks, leg-outs, one-legged leg lifts,
and vertical scissors

Side leg lifts

Marching in place on toes

All variations of push-ups

Chin-ups, pull-ups

Dips

If overweight, fast walking or slow jogging with no incline or hills

If not overweight, all or any upper-body exercises with moderate to
heavy weights and dead lifts with no weight

* PLEASE NOTE: THE PRECEDING EXERCISES ARE RECOMMENDED FOR SPOONS. REMEM-
BER THAT *NO ONE* EXERCISE CAN BRING TRUE FITNESS. YOU NEED TO PERFORM A
FULL-BODY EXERCISE ROUTINE EACH AND EVERY TIME YOU WORK OUT. MAKE SURE
THAT YOUR FITNESS REGIMEN IS MADE UP OF THE EXERCISES LISTED ABOVE. (SEE
CHAPTER 8 FOR SPOON WORKOUT ROUTINES AND INSTRUCTIONS ON HOW TO BEST
PERFORM THE SUGGESTED EXERCISES.)

Exercises to Avoid if You Want
to Escape Your Spoon Shape

Squats

Lunges

Leg presses

Leg extensions and leg curls

Ankle weights

All elliptical machines

All stair climbers/steppers

All step classes

Versa climbers

Long-distance running at high speeds

Sprinting

Roller blading

Sliding

Skating

Swimming

Kick-boxing

Spinning

All high-impact aerobic and exercise classes

All lower-body exercises with moderate to high resistance or weights

Walking or jogging on any sort of incline

Rowing with lower-body resistance

Jumping rope with a weighted rope

Inner-outer leg machines

Cross-country ski machine with lower-body resistance

Summary

As a Spoon, the rule of thumb is high reps and low resistance for *all* lower-body exercises, and moderate to high resistance for all upper-body exercises. If you're overweight, the resistance should not be too high for the upper body. You don't want to push out the fat as you build muscle underneath. Until you are at a weight and size you're happy with, do not increase the resistance or weight on any exercise, but rather increase the frequency and number of repetitions to continue to burn off fat and inches.

THE RULER PROFILE

Most Rulers are fortunate when it comes to finding clothes that fit. They are similar to Hourglasses in that their bodies are pretty much in proportion, but they are not as tapered in the midsection, with no significant difference between the sizes of their chest, waist and hips. They're built straight up and down. Fashion and runway models examplify skinny Rulers. Rulers tend to carry excess weight on their stomachs and butts. They don't get wider, but rather protrude fore and aft. When a Ruler gains 10 pounds, it is very visible. Most Rulers have small to medium frames and do not possess a lot of muscle mass, hence their need to keep their weight lower than any other body types. Typically, Rulers bulk the least of any body type, and if not overweight, can perform virtually any exercise without the fear of unwanted mass in any region of their bodies. Rulers, however, possess less strength and need to work out extra hard to build muscle, strength and power. Although most Rulers are small to medium chested, occasionally you'll find a woman Ruler with big breasts. It is imperative for those women to perform a lot of upper-body and abdominal exercises to help support the back, shoulders and arms in order to avoid poor posture and hunching. Rulers give the appearance of being "thin." And on a scale they tend to weight even less than they appear to. Rulers also may tend to be underweight and overfat, which means they may be carrying too much body fat and not enough lean mass (muscle).

Problem Areas and Characteristics

Rulers are fortunate in the sense that if they're not overweight, they do not have to work out as often as the other body types. Losing weight or mass requires frequent exercise; changing your shape does not. The typical Ruler needs to work out no more than 3 days per week to change his or her body. But he or she needs to exercise intensely, really taxing the muscles. Because the Ruler's workout is typically more anaerobic than aerobic, more rest is required between these intense workouts. Rulers make the best joggers and long-distance runners because of the way their mass is distributed over their frames. They simply put less stress on their joints. They also excel in any movements or sports that require long and sustained aerobic actions. Have you ever seen a world-class Cone, Spoon or heavy-Hourglass long-distance runner or swimmer? Of course not, and now you know why. On the other hand, because it is more difficult for Rulers to build mass, you don't see professional Ruler bodybuilders.

Often, because of their poor hamstring flexibility and weak lower abs, Rulers experience lower back pain. As they age, their bones and joints are more susceptible to osteoporosis and bone fractures than other body types. Because Rulers need to work extra hard to build muscle mass, it's vital that they do not allow that muscle mass to fade. In fact, Rulers generally have no problem losing mass throughout their upper and lower bodies (unlike Hourglasses, who need to work hard at it).

Of all the body types, Rulers seem to exercise the least. Perhaps because many Rulers are "naturally thin," they feel they can get away without exercising. It is quite common for Rulers reaching their 40s and 50s to suddenly gain a lot of weight, especially in their midsection. And because they've often been inactive for most of their lives, they have a hard time adjusting psychologically to the fact that they need to exercise regularly. Most men are Rulers and should focus on trimming their midsection and increasing hamstring flexibility to avoid back problems later in life.

Best Exercises for Escaping Your Ruler Shape*

Unless you're overweight, all of these exercises are recommended. If you need to reduce your weight, use light to moderate resistance and weights until you reach your ideal weight.

Stretching, especially hamstring and quadricep muscle groups

Full sit-ups without locking feet, upper and lower abdominal crunches, and leg-outs

Step classes

Spinning

Squats, lunges, and leg presses with moderate to high weights

Hand and ankle weights

Stationary biking with moderate to high resistance

Walking, jogging or running on an incline or on hills

All ellipitical machines with moderate to high resistance

Stepper/stair climbers with moderate to high resistance

Push-ups

Chin-ups, pull-ups

Dips

Chair push-ups and introverted push-ups

Sprinting

Water aerobics

Swimming

Ski machines with resistance for both upper and lower bodies

Roller blading on hills

Kick-boxing

Jumping rope with a peg or weighted rope

Inner-outer leg machines with moderate to high weights

Rowing with moderate to high resistance for both upper and lower bodies

All upper- or lower-body exercises using moderate to high resistance or weights

* PLEASE NOTE: THE PRECEDING EXERCISES ARE RECOMMENDED FOR RULERS. REMEMBER THAT *NO ONE* EXERCISE CAN BRING TRUE FITNESS. YOU NEED TO PERFORM A FULL-BODY EXERCISE ROUTINE EACH AND EVERY TIME YOU WORK OUT. MAKE SURE THAT YOUR FITNESS REGIMEN IS MADE UP OF THE EXERCISES LISTED ABOVE. (SEE CHAPTER 9 FOR RULER WORKOUT ROUTINES AND INSTRUCTIONS ON HOW TO BEST PERFORM THE SUGGESTED EXERCISES.)

Exercises to Avoid if You Want to Escape Your Ruler Shape*

None

* PLEASE NOTE: ALTHOUGH THERE ARE NO EXERCISES TO AVOID UNLESS YOU ARE AN OVERWEIGHT RULER, SOME ABDOMINAL AND LEG EXERCISES MAY CAUSE SOME DISCOMFORT TO THE LOWER BACK REGION. AS YOUR HAMSTRING FLEXIBILITY AND ABDOMINAL STRENGTH INCREASE, YOU MAY BEGIN TO *ADD* EXERCISES FROM THE FOLLOWING LIST TO YOUR REGIMEN.

Vertical scissors
One-legged leg lifts
Side leg lifts
Dead lifts
Leg lifts

Summary

As a Ruler, you pretty much have free rein to perform any kind of exercise provided you are not overweight. If you are overweight, ease up on the weights and resistance a little bit until you start to trim down. Then you can incorporate both. Protect your back! Don't skip your stretching routine before you work out and stretch your hamstrings lightly at the end of all of your workouts. Focus on increasing the intensity of each exercise and to prevent injury pay careful attention to your form and body alignment. Do your abdominal work in the beginning of your workouts when your motivation and energy is highest to ensure that you do it every time.

THE CONE PROFILE

While only 10 percent of women are Cones, the same body type describes 30 percent of all men. Cone men, especially those who exercise with weights, generally look out of proportion because they neglect their lower bodies. Cones are the polar opposite of Spoons. Their upper bodies are considerably larger and stronger than their lower bodies. Typically, a female Cone's best asset is her legs while a male Cone's is his chest. Miniskirts are a must for Cone women because they draw the viewer's eyes away from the breasts and stomach. Usually short-waisted and long-legged, Cones benefit from abundant aerobic exercise combined with abdominal and upper-body endurance exercises, which are crucial. They strengthen and protect the back and shoulder regions. Overweight cones look even more so because most of that extra weight is concentrated on top. That, of course, creates an even greater disparity between the upper and lower bodies. Cones have a propensity for tight hamstrings (just as Rulers do) and their abdominals are usually weak because Cones don't typically work on this region. They tend to look shorter than they actually are, especially when overweight. Cone women who slim down their upper bodies, especially their abdominals, will start to look more like Hourglasses. A typical female Cone's measurements are 40-35-32. With proper exercise, that cone woman could be 36-30-32.

Problem Areas and Characteristics

Cones carry a lot of weight and mass in their upper back and chest. Their arms are usually large as well, and have excess fat, especially on the backs of the arms (triceps). Their stomachs usually protrude, an unwanted natural tendency that is especially noticeable in both men and women. As they grow older, their posture seems to worsen unless they strengthen their abdominals and increase their hamstring flexibility. Movements or sports that require upper-body power and speed—such as racquet sports and track events including the javelin throw, discuss and shot-put—come easily to most Cones. Any sport that requires quick and short movements and requires upper-body strength is agreeable to Cones, whereas jogging or running for long distances can be very uncomfortable. I find that most Cone women are very self-conscious of people leering at their upper bodies when they do any kind of impact sports or activities. Male Cones who frequent the gym look very out of proportion. Most need to switch from heavy weights to much lighter ones when they work out and focus more on their lower bodies. Cones who exercise rarely develop osteoporosis in their upper bodies, but because they are more susceptible to lower-body injuries, especially hip fractures, it's important to strengthen and add some mass to their lower bodies as a preventative measure.

Most important to protect is the upper and lower back. This can be accomplished through weight loss on top and lots of stretching and abdominal exercises.

Best Exercises for Escaping Your Cone Shape*

Spinning
Squats
Lunges
Leg presses
Leg extensions and leg curls
Stepper/stair climbers
Stationary biking with moderate to high resistance
Full sit-ups, leg-outs, and upper and lower abdominal crunches
Hamstring stretches
Upper-body stretches
Jumping rope with a speed rope
Dead lifts
Kick-boxing using lower body only
Ankle weights
Low-impact step classes
Ski machines with light tension for upper body and moderate to high resistance for lower body
All lower-body exercises using moderate to high resistance or weights
Slow walking on an incline or on hills
Inner-outer thigh machines with moderate to heavy weights

* PLEASE NOTE: THE PRECEDING EXERCISES ARE RECOMMENDED FOR CONES. REMEMBER THAT NO ONE EXERCISE CAN BRING TRUE FITNESS. YOU NEED TO PERFORM A FULL-BODY EXERCISE ROUTINE EACH AND EVERY TIME YOU WORK OUT. MAKE SURE THAT YOUR FITNESS REGIMEN IS MADE UP OF THE EXERCISES LISTED ABOVE. (SEE CHAPTER 10 FOR CONE WORKOUT ROUTINES AND INSTRUCTIONS ON HOW TO BEST PERFORM THE SUGGESTED EXERCISES.)

Exercises to Avoid if You Want to Escape Your Cone Shape

Bench press with moderate to heavy weights
Decline push-ups
Triceps kick-backs with moderate to heavy weights
Triceps extensions with moderate to heavy weights
Hand weights
Rowing
All upper-body exercises with moderate to heavy resistance or weights
Aerobic and exercise classes that use Heavy Hands or weights
Kick-boxing classes using upper-body movements
Jumping rope with a weighted rope

Summary

As a Cone, the rule of thumb is high reps and low resistance or weights for the upper body and high resistance and moderate to heavy weights for the lower body. Although unusual, a few Cones may bulk down below a bit if they are overweight. Typically, Cones shy away from abdominal exercises and lower-body exercises. It's important to focus on these areas so the body becomes better proportioned. Cones, especially male Cones, have a harder time than other body types giving up the heavy weight lifting for their upper bodies. I suggest switching to more natural exercises such as push-ups, dips, chin-ups, or upper-body exercise routines with low weights and higher repetitions. You'll still possess great upper-body strength and your body will look much better proportioned.

BODY TYPE AND AEROBIC FITNESS EQUIPMENT CHART

	SPOON	HOURGLASS	RULER	CONE
Stationary bike	✳ Use light tension/ high RPMs.	✳ Use light tension/ high RPMs.	● Use tension.	● Use tension.
Treadmill	✳ Fast walking with no incline is okay. Never use an incline.	✳ Fast walking or running with no incline is okay. Never use an incline.	✳ Use an incline to walk or run.	✳ Use an incline to walk or run.
Stair climbers	NR	NR	●	●
Rower	●	✳ Use light resistance.	●	✳ Use light resistance.
Ski machine	✳ Use light resistance for lower body, high resistance for upper body.	✳ Use light resistance for lower body and upper body.	✳ Use resistance for upper and lower body.	✳ Use high resistance for lower body, light resistance for upper body.
Aerobic riders (HealthRider)	✳ Use light resistance.	✳ Use light resistance.	●	✳ Use light resistance.
Jump rope	●	●	✳ May use weighted jump rope.	●
Spinning Ellipticals Stair climbers Versa climbers Step	NR	NR	● Use resistance.	✳ Use resistance for lower body. Do not use hand weights or resistance for upper body.

NR = Not recommended for this body type

● = Yes

✳ = Yes, with specific instructions

## CHAPTER 3

Your Fitness Checklist

Now that you know your body type and understand its importance in achieving your fitness and aesthetic goals, you are ready to start planning your customized fitness routine. As I often tell my clients, performing the exercises necessary to escape your shape is the easy part. What's far more laborious is organizing your life and creating a *clear* path for fitness within it. You must be able to exercise consistently despite any constraint. This chapter will serve as a roadmap and checklist that will safeguard your steps to starting and maintaining a consistent workout schedule. It doesn't matter how effective or great *any* exercise regimen is, if you cannot perform it regularly, you will never escape your shape. Keep that in mind: consistency is the most important element of *every* fitness regimen.

BEFORE YOU START EXERCISING
Get a Physical

Everyone over 25 years of age, especially those who are not presently exercising *vigorously,* should get a full physical and stress test. No exceptions! I'm shocked at the number of people who come to me who have not had a full physical for years. There are many sound reasons for getting a physical, but I've found the best motivator for those who don't regularly get checkups is this thought: God forbid you develop a disease or condition that lingers or worsens for years before you do anything about it. You could be whittling away your chances of survival by avoiding the doctor. On the other hand, had you received a physical each year and had you contracted something, it could have been addressed and treated immediately. Early detection is the key to full recovery from most ailments. So, please, get a physical!

Another excellent reason to get a physical, particularly if you've been sedentary, is that your doctor can advise you where to begin in terms of workout intensity. Even if you're in "good health," your heart rate is not used to jumping from your standing pulse to the upper portion of your training zone. Ex-athletes who were once in fine shape but for the last ten years have been sitting at a desk cannot and should not start exercising where they left off a decade before. It would put them at high risk for injury or even a heart attack. So, for all of you who have not performed a full-body exercise routine within the last year, please start out slowly. In a few short weeks, you'll be able to increase your intensity and the duration of your workouts. For those of you with special medical conditions, I strongly advise that you seek professional help before you begin to exercise unless you are confident and knowledgeable that you know what you're doing. There's no point in exercising vigorously if it only exacerbates a condition.

Assess Your Lifestyle

The purpose of this section is to get you to make an honest evaluation of your lifestyle so that no matter what fate pushes in your path, you can always make time for exercise. From time to time, your schedule will change. Life will throw a curveball and suddenly your waking hours scheduled so neatly are thrown into chaos. Anticipating certain lifestyle constraints means formulating a Plan B, a way to stick to your plan to work out three times a week, for example, even if the alarm doesn't go off, if you have to travel out of town unexpectedly, if your child takes ill, or whatever. Assessing your lifestyle will help you choose *where, when* and *how long* you need to be exercising to reach your goals.

First let's look at what happens when you aren't honest with yourself. Mary came to my office unhappy with her body. She's an Hourglass, weighs 160 pounds and wears a size 12. She would like to lose about 10 pounds and drop down to a size 8. "I've been working out for years!" Mary claims, with nothing to show for it. I ask for more information about her current fitness routine and learn that she belongs to a health club where she says she does "a lot of cardio" and has also tried various exercise classes, running, biking, and the StairMaster. Nothing works. These figures just aren't adding up, so I probe a little deeper and ask when she has time for the gym. She tries to get there in the evenings, but rarely makes it. She has to get the kids off to school in the morning, so that's no good, and her weekends are full of carpools and social events so that by the end of the day she's exhausted. Now we're getting somewhere.

"Come on, Mary," I prod, "tell me honestly. How many times in an average week do you make it to the gym?"

She pauses, then whispers shamefully, "Two. . . . Well, actually, Wednesdays my husband has the kids so I can usually make it there on Wednesday." In a few minutes Mary went from a devoted and disciplined exerciser to a woman who works out once a week at best. She's active all right, but lacking the consistency that is the key to a successful fitness plan. Even if it's only 40 minutes, 3 days a week. If you stick to that week in and week out, and perform the right exercises for your body type, then you will see change. I challenged Mary, and I challenge you to take an honest look at your behavior. What kind of effort are you really making. What can you actually commit to?

Take a realistic look at your life and think about how your work schedule, family and other commitments can and do conflict with your exercise plans, so that you can find solutions and ultimately be successful. This is just as important as determining your body type and following the appropriate workout. In order to escape your shape, you need to be consistent. The goal is to organize and prioritize your time so that working out becomes a habit, not an afterthought. If you are just starting or are inconsistent with your workouts, you need to ask yourself these questions:

How much time do I spend at work? How many hours and on what days?

How long does it take me to get to and from work?

How often do I travel? Is it for work or pleasure?

Can I get to the gym on a consistent basis? Is it open when I have time to exercise?

Am I better off working out at home?

Who can I enlist to watch the kids while I'm exercising?

The answers to these questions will help determine where you should be exercising, on which days and for how long. Fortunately, there is not a lot of fitness equipment or space required in order for you to perform *any* of the body-type workouts.

ON THE ROAD

Many of my clients complain that their busy travel schedules get in the way of their workouts. While they're at home, things are dandy, but as soon as they hit the road, it all falls to pieces. Part of the problem is that they don't find the equipment they use at their health club in hotel gyms. So they seesaw between weeks of terrific workouts and frustrating weeks of inaction. If you have a busy travel schedule, don't be frustrated that the hotels you stay in don't feature the same facilities your health club does. Most hotels just don't have the space to house lots of elaborate equipment. Instead, you need to devise a routine that is less dependent on machines.

It's equally important that you practice your road routine before you go away. Don't wait until you're in a hotel to try out your new routine. Testing it out beforehand will serve you well: You'll know exactly how long it's going to take to complete the entire workout, so you can make adjustments if necessary. You'll get used to working out without machines. You'll become familiar with the routine and know exactly what do to.

Instead of focusing on what you "can't do," focus your energy on what you can control. In this case, since the hotels you'll be staying at probably won't offer the same equipment your gym does, prepare yourself, both mentally and physically. For starters incorporate a jump rope into your routine and bring it along. It's great aerobic and toning exercise and you can bring it with you anywhere. You can get an effective workout on the road and stop your stop-start exercising.

BLOCKING OUT THE TIME

You need only an hour 3 to 5 days a week to commit to this program. If you cannot block that much time, you can split up your workouts into two half-hour time slots, but it's far simpler to do it all at once. Changing clothes, not to mention gears, takes time too, after all, but if you don't have any alternative, then do whatever it takes in order to regularly complete your fitness regimen. If you currently belong to a gym or are thinking of joining one, consider how long it takes to get there. If it takes more than 15 or 20 minutes whether you're walking or driving, don't join. Unless you have a very relaxed schedule and virtually no other responsibilities other than taking care of yourself, the commute alone may prevent you from sticking to your exercise plan. Why? 20 minutes to get there, 60 minutes to exercise, 20 minutes to shower and dress and 20 minutes to get home

equals 2 hours. Most people do not have 2 hours a day to allo-
cate to their fitness cause. That's one of the reasons why only 2
out of 10 people who join health clubs use them as often as
twice a week. The minute a stressor or change in your personal
or professional life occurs, the first thing that suffers is your
workouts. If you find yourself in this predicament, then you
need to think about purchasing some fitness equipment and
doing your workouts at home. If you can afford it, you might
decide to do both.

I'm often asked whether it is better to work out in the morning or evening. The truth is, there is little medical evidence to
suggest that either is more beneficial. Whenever your schedule
allows you 45 to 60 uninterrupted minutes is the best time for
you to be exercising. Try to exercise at the same time on each of
your workout days. The reason is that your body will grow accustomed to it, just as you're used to eating and sleeping at regular intervals during the course of your 24-hour day. Sometimes
the time slot you allot for exercise is not ideal for you. For example, you may enjoy working out in the morning because your
energy is highest then, but you just can't squeeze in a morning
workout. If it's too difficult to match your preferences with
your hectic schedule, over time your body will adjust to the
time that does fit in.

I find that when I perform high-intensity anaerobic exercises
such as chin-ups, dips, and push-ups in the early morning, I feel
tired the rest of the day. But when I limit my morning exercise
to aerobic activities such as biking or jumping rope, I feel energized throughout the day. The reason, I believe, is that after
many hours of sleep, your body and heart rate are sluggish.
Anaerobic exercise is a shock to your system. Your heart rate
soars when you lift weights, for example, considerably higher
than when you jog. So, if you need to work out in the early
morning and will be doing anaerobic exercise, a longer warmup
(more than 15 minutes) will cushion the shock to your system.
For those of you who need to split up your workout, try to do

your aerobic portion in the morning and anaerobic portion later in the day. Some of my clients tell me that at the end of a work day they're so exhausted that the last thing they want to do is work out. If that sounds familiar, you need to ask yourself if your fatigue is psychological or physical. If you had a good night's sleep and a grueling day at work, it's the former. You should work out as vigorously as possible. But if, on the other hand, you had very little sleep, it's physical and you should exercise only mildly. You don't want to risk injuring yourself during your workout. When you're mentally fatigued and really don't feel like exercising, push through it and get on that bike or treadmill. Once you start moving and break a sweat, your body will begin to wake up. Before you know it, you'll be halfway through your workout. Overcoming that feeling is something you learn to do. You need to remind yourself each time you're tired and don't feel like working out that the last time you felt that way and worked out anyway, you felt much better afterward. Focus on just getting on that bike or treadmill, and you'll be on your way to maintaining consistency!

When all is said and done, finding time to exercise boils down to priorities. How important is it to you? How much do you value fitness? Are you willing to sacrifice some of your idle time and apply it constructively? The more you see your body change for the better, the more time you will find for fitness. By exercising based on your body type, you will see your body reshape quickly and your motivation to exercise—even when you think you don't have time—will not get in the way of your becoming and staying fit for the rest of your life.

CONSIDER YOUR MEDICAL AND ORTHOPEDIC BACKGROUND

Your medical and orthopedic background dictates which exercises you should avoid. In fact, it is the only factor that takes precedent over your body type when choosing the type of exercises you will be performing. For instance, if you're a Ruler with a severe disc problem in your lower back, you'll want to avoid running, even though it is a recommended exercise for your body type. You would do far better with a recumbent bike (that would protect your back) as your primary aerobic activity. Too often, people either do not go to a specialist for exercise dos and don'ts *prior* to engaging in a fitness regimen or they ignore a serious condition thinking that it will go away with time. Among my clients, joggers with foot and leg problems are the worst offenders. If you're injured, you cannot exercise regularly. And if you cannot exercise on a consistent basis, you cannot change or even maintain your fitness level. So get smart and do the right thing for your body. I'm amazed when runners flatly refuse to switch over to biking because they can't get the same "high." To that I say you'll get a better high from biking than sitting, resting and icing your body back into fighting form.

Fear of injury is the number one reason why the elderly do not exercise. I wish I had a dollar for every time I've heard someone say, "I'm scared to start an exercise program. I'm forty pounds overweight, seventy years old, have a bad back, achy knees and arthritis. Besides, what good will it do me now? I'll never be able to get in shape." Excess weight and medical and orthopedic constraints are not acceptable excuses for not exercising. In fact, they're good reasons to start a fitness regimen. One of the great things about proper exercise is that after working out for just a few months, your body will respond as if you'd been working out all your life. You're never too old to start or to realize the benefits of exercising. And if you want to live to a ripe old age, I strongly suggest you start now. Too often, people are either misinformed or lack the self-confidence to do it. The key is to begin slowly and ease into your formal routine. Riding a recumbent stationary bike (one that has a chairlike seat), for 10 to 20 minutes at low resistance, then stretching for a couple of minutes is a good start. Once you build up some cardiovascular conditioning, you can add some other exercises. Don't worry about how your progress compares to anyone else's—the road to fitness is an individual journey. Your job is to align yourself with positive influences that will support you in your endeavor. If your medical condition is serious and chronic, I suggest you contact your local hospital's rehabilitation center and ask around for an exercise specialist to help get you going.

Aside from the health benefits, the purpose of fitness is to enable us to enjoy our lives and embrace whichever physical activities lend meaning and purpose to us. The person who refuses to exercise because of an injury is really saying, "I don't know how to exercise around my physical constraints." In all my years and expertise in this field I *never* once met an individual who did not benefit from proper and regular exercise. With time and perseverance you will be able to intensify your workouts, adding exercises to your regime that you once thought impossible. Sometimes you need to walk before you can run. Don't be discouraged because you cannot do everything you desire exercise-wise on day one. That's no excuse not to start.

Here's a good rule to follow while exercising: if it hurts, STOP! There are so many factors that determine how your body will react to a particular exercise. They include how athletic or active you were as a child, how many years you've been exercising, how intensely you exercise, and your flexibility as well as your mental toughness. If you do develop a physical constraint that prevents you from sticking with a tried-and-true regime, you'll need to learn to work around it. The key to maintaining your fitness level and mental stimulation is substituting that particular exercise with another that will not stress your injured area. I was once partial to running, but as a child had a number of ankle and leg fractures. So instead of running 3 or 4 days per week and stressing my body, I jump rope instead. When my body feels strong, I go for the occasional run, but never more than once or twice a week because I know that it will put undue stress on my body. Then I'll have to rest for days, abstaining from lower-body exercises. In other words, the risk isn't worth the benefit. For those of you with chronic lower-body aches and pains who are just starting out, try a stationary bike—I find it the most effective and least stressful form of aerobic exercise.

CALCULATE YOUR
TARGET HEART RATE (THR) ZONE

The intensity of your workout—how hard you're working—can make or break your fitness program. The easiest way for you to measure intensity is by checking your heart rate *during* a fitness session, that is, the number of times your heart beats in a minute. As you get in better shape, heart rate and target heart zone will increase because you'll be able to work harder without straining your heart. The more fit you become, the stronger your heart becomes. Even as you move into your 60s, 70s and 80s, you can continue to strengthen your heart with consistent and proper exercise, though as you age, your target heart rate decreases.

Your target heart rate (THR) is defined as the heart rate recommended during vigorous exercise for your age and fitness level. When you're in your target heart rate zone, it means you're exercising with the proper intensity. Exercising above your THR means you're exercising too vigorously; exercising below your THR, or under your zone, means you're not exercising vigorously enough. How hard should you work during exercise? The answer depends on several factors, but the threshold needed to achieve health benefits is lower for those who are sedentary than for those who are very fit (see the Exer-Form Chart, page 68). Your age, primary risk factors for heart disease, high blood pressure, family history of heart disease, and stress levels, among others, dictate where you should begin.

To determine your heart rate zone, follow these steps:

1. First subtract your age from 220. This number represents your maximal heart rate. For example, a 50-year-old woman has a maximal heart rate of 170 (220 − 50 = 170). Her heart

rate should not exceed 170 beats per minute during any type of physical activity. There are a few exceptions. For instance, professional or well-trained athletes may exceed that intensity. But most of you should monitor your heart rate during exercise in part to avoid overexerting yourself (see page 62).

2. To calculate the low end of your zone, multiply you maximal heart rate by .6. For our 50-year-old woman, that would be 170 × .60 = 102. That means in order to gain some benefits from her regime, she must work hard enough for her heart to beat at least 102 times per minute.

3. Calculate the high end of your zone by multiplying your maximal heart rate by .75. Our 50-year-old woman's is 170 × .75 = 128. So a 50-year-old semifit woman whose goal is to lose weight should be exercising just hard enough for the heart to beat between 102 and 128 beats per minute.

How will your heart react when you begin or intensify your exercise program? That depends on how fit you are. The risk of heart problems is higher for sedentary people than for those who are more active. If you're a very active person, your heart is used to being taxed, though that's not to say an active lifestyle can substitute for a fitness program.

Most people start out with a program that's either under or over their zone. And very few warm up or stretch prior to increasing the intensity (energy) level. Remember, your heart rate jumps faster with anaerobic exercises than with aerobic ones. So use your THR zone as a guideline, then monitor your heart rate during exercise (see Gauge the Intensity of Your Workout, below) since your heart rate increases as you increase the intensity of your activity.

GAUGE THE INTENSITY OF YOUR WORKOUT

When you embark on a new exercise program, your heart rate should linger in the low end of your heart rate zone. I strongly recommend that anyone over 35 years of age get a stress test done prior to engaging in any exercise or activity that causes their heart rate to go from a standing pulse (resting heart rate) to 70 percent of their maximal heart rate. This, by the way, includes most exercises recommended in Part Two.

Checking Your Heart Rate During Exercise

It's important to know your target zone before you begin exercising. (If you haven't done so already, see page 60 on how to do it.)

To monitor your heart rate during your workout:

- Stop whatever you're doing and within 3 seconds locate your pulse at your neck, wrist, or temple with the tips of your index and middle fingers. Don't use your thumb, which has a pulse of its own. If taking your pulse on your chest, place the heel of your right hand over your heart.
- Use a clock with a second hand to count the number of beats for 6 seconds.
- Multiply that number by 10 to calculate your heart rate.

    That number represents how many times your heart is beating per minute during that particular exercise. If you're not in your zone, adjust your intensity level by either raising or lowering the intensity.

Take your pulse every 5 to 10 minutes during your workout. With practice you won't have to check your pulse so often. You'll simply feel and know how hard you're working. If you experience shortness of breath, find that you're not able to talk comfortably during aerobic exercise or are feeling dizzy or nauseous, stop exercising *immediately,* place a wet, cool towel on your head and lie down on your back, feet level with your head.

When starting out, it's more important to increase the time you spend exercising than the intensity. Begin with low-intensity exercises, such as riding a stationary bike with light resistance or walking slowly on a treadmill. Remember that the more risk factors you have, the more critical it is for you to exercise closer to the low end or even under the low end of your zone. Your zone is only a range and a guide to follow. If you are exercising and find that you're huffing and puffing, check your pulse. If you are still under your zone, decrease the intensity level immediately. Even though you're under your prescribed zone, you are still getting benefits from the exercise. With time, you will be able to exercise comfortably within your zone, and you'll even have to increase it. Don't get discouraged.

Use your heart rate to monitor your progress. I highly recommend heart-rate monitors for people with a heart complication. You strap this nifty device around your chest and it provides continuous feedback on how hard your heart is working. Heart monitors make it easy to see if you are about to go above or below your zone, so you can adjust the intensity of your exertions accordingly. While I've worked with countless people with heart conditions, I'm not a physician. A doctor's care and the monitoring of your heart rate during exercising are musts for all heart condition patients.

Remaining in your zone during your workout is important, but doesn't necessarily mean you are becoming more fit or that your body will change in the areas that you expect it to. Many people who come to me for help exercise consistently within their target zones, but do the wrong type of exercise for their body type. For example, if you have a Spoon-shaped body and are using step classes as your primary means of exercise, you'll never change your body to your desired level of satisfaction. Sure, you'll become a little more fit, but if you can become more fit and mold your body to your ideal at the same time, why not?

RATINGS OF PERCEIVED EXERTION (RPE)

Another popular means of measuring intensity during exercise is with the "perceived exertion" scale. Rather than using a formula, Borg's scale, also known as the Ratings of Perceived Exertion (RPE), was developed to allow exercisers to subjectively rate their feelings during exercise, taking into account personal fitness level, environmental conditions and general fatigue. Currently, two RPE scales are widely used, the original which rates exercise intensity on a scale of 6 to 20, and the revised scale on which you can rate exertion from 0 to 10. I use the revised scale with my clients because the terminology is easier to understand, though both account for the increase in heart rate during exercise.

You don't have to be quick with numbers to use the Borg scale. While exercising, you simply ask yourself, "How hard am I exerting myself?" and assign a number value to your answer. The low end of the scale (0) means you're not exerting yourself at all. The high end of the scale (10) represents the point at which you could push yourself no harder. If you feel that you are at a 3, then based on your medical background and unique

REVISED SCALE FOR RATINGS OF PERCEIVED EXERTION (RPE)

0	Nothing at all
0.5	Very, very weak
1	Very weak
2	Weak
3	Moderate
4	Somewhat strong
5	Strong
6	
7	Very strong
8	
9	
10	Very, very strong
—	Maximal

TAKEN FROM *ACSM's GUIDELINES FOR EXERCISE TESTING AND PRESCRIPTION*, 5TH ED., 1995.

constraints, you can either pick up intensity or lower it. After rating your exertion, you may want to take your pulse. It should fall somewhere in the zone that you've chosen according to your goals. I highly recommend this scale for healthy individuals. For those with heart problems or other special constraints, I recommend using a heart-rate monitor to ensure your safety.

TRAINING HEART RATE ZONE

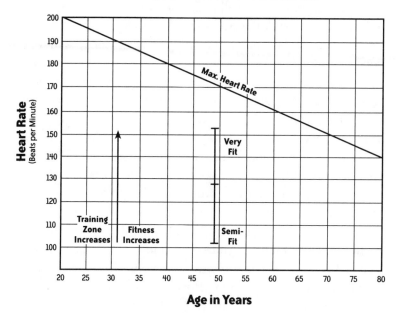

Examples

A 50-year-old semifit Individual (see the Exer-Form Chart, page 68)

$220 - 50 = 170$ Maximum Heart Rate

Low End = $.60 \times 170 = 102$ THR

High End = $.75 \times 170 = 128$ THR

A 50-year-old very fit individual

Low End = $.75 \times 170 = 128$ THR

High End = $.90 \times 170 = 153$ THR

DECIDING WHAT YOU WANT
OUT OF YOUR FITNESS PROGRAM

Whether you want to exercise for overall health, to lose weight, to build muscle mass, to enhance your sports performance or simply to firm up, you still must make time for exercise and make the right fitness choices before you begin. Often, the folks who come to see me haven't accomplished what they set out to do because they didn't do all their homework first. For instance, let's say you enjoy skiing. You've booked a January trip but your fall schedule is beyond hectic. Work takes priority and your good intentions to shape up for the trip take a backseat. Before you know it, December is upon you. Suddenly you're frantic to "get in shape." You start working out 3 or 4 days per week but before the second week is out, you overdo it and injure yourself. That's no way to start the ski season.

My recommendation is that ski nuts exercise 2 or 3 days per week year-round. They manage to find time to exercise when the ski season is upon them, why not before? The good news is that skiers (and they're not alone) have something to motivate them—and nonskiers can find that something, too. It doesn't matter how you motivate yourself, as long as you can sustain it. The difficult part is being *honest* with yourself so that your expectations are based on the effort you're willing to put in. I often strike a chord with my clients by asking them how successful they would be at work if they devoted a single day a week to it. Obviously, working one day a week won't get you to the corner office. Or how about reading to your child only once a week, would he/she grow up to be good at reading? Probably not. Well, the same is true for an exercise regime. If you choose to exercise just once or twice a week, that's okay. But don't expect dramatic changes or complain that you hate the way you look and feel. You haven't earned the right to look great.

I can't count the number of men who come to me for advice who have a clear idea of the way they want to look but can't commit to the devotion it requires. They want to develop bigger muscles, especially in their chests and arms. They've bought weight-gain supplements and joined gyms where they work out for a couple of hours a day, 6 days per week. At least they do at first. But after the first month, work and other commitments start taking priority over gym time. Before they know it, they're visiting the gym 1 or 2 days a week, mostly on the weekends.

The truth is, these guys never had a chance to succeed—not because they lacked physical ability, but because their time-consuming approach to fitness didn't fit into their busy lifestyles. The first thing these guys need to understand is that they didn't fail. Their plans did. They *can* get bigger. But they need a different routine—one that consists of four 1-hour work-outs per week, a routine that they can do until they're 80 or older. The *key* question you need to ask yourself when access-ing your goals and deciding what you want out of your fitness regimen is, Will I be able to do most of the exercises I'm cur-rently performing 2, 5, 10 years from now? Of course you may need to make minor adjustments along the way. But reaching your goals has more to do with the planning you do *before* you set out than with the act of exercising itself!

THE EXER-FORM CHART

The most difficult thing to figure out is the percentage of aerobic vs. anaerobic exercise necessary to achieve both your weight-loss and toning goals. Aerobic exercises are primarily used for weight loss; anaerobic exercises are better suited for toning the body. That said, it's imperative to know and follow certain prin-ciples so that (a) your body changes for the better and (b) your motivation remains high so that you continue to work out regu-larly.

The function of the Exer-Form Chart is to help guide you in choosing the right mix of frequency (how often you exercise), duration (how long you exercise for each period), intensity

EXER-FORM CHART

Principles

Goals	FREQUENCY (Days per week)	DURATION (How long of a period)	INTENSITY (How hard you're working/THR)	TYPE (Aerobic/anaerobic amount of time)
Weight Loss (For Sedentary Individual)	4–6 days per week	30–45 minutes	Low (THR 50%–60%)	90% aerobic 10% anaerobic first 3 months 80% aerobic 20% anaerobic after 3 months
Toning (For Sedentary Individual)	2–3 days per week	20–30 minutes	Low (THR 55%–70%)	60% aerobic 40% anaerobic first 3 months 50% aerobic 50% anaerobic after 3 months
Weight Loss (For Active/ Semi-Fit)	4–6 days per week	40–60 minutes	Moderate (THR 50%–75%)	80% aerobic 20% anaerobic first 3 months 70% aerobic 30% anaerobic after 3 months
Toning (For Active/ Semi-Fit)	2–4 days per week	30–45 minutes	Moderate (THR 65%–80%)	50% aerobic 50% anaerobic first 3 months 40% aerobic 60% anaerobic after 3 months
Weight Loss (For Very Active/ Very Fit)	4–6 days per week	60–75 minutes	High (THR 75%–90%)	70% aerobic 30% anaerobic first 3 months 60% aerobic 40% anaerobic after 3 months
Toning (For Very Active/ Very Fit)	3–4 days per week	60–75 minutes	High (THR 80%–95%)	40% aerobic 60% anaerobic first 3 months 30% aerobic 70% anaerobic after 3 months

(how hard you work out) and exercise type (aerobic vs. anaerobic). Based on your current level of fitness, you match up your goals (weight loss or toning) and follow the prescribed formula. These formulas work for all body types though your type dictates what kind of aerobic and anaerobic exercises you should be performing (see Part Two for exercises suited to your body type). As you increase your fitness level, you should adjust your formula—moving down the chart. In effect, adjusting your formula means increasing your *intensity* as you become more fit. If you find yourself losing more weight and mass than you intended, you should adjust to increase the proportion of anaerobic exercises in your workout. Conversely, if you are not losing the weight or mass you'd hoped to, you need to increase the proportion of aerobic exercise in your routine until your body starts to change in that direction.

IN REVIEW

Here's a checklist for you to look at to make sure you're prepared to move forward.

Have you:

✓ *Received a full physical?*

✓ *Assessed your lifestyle, made time for your fitness goals and determined where you'll be working out, on which days and for how long?*

✓ *Taken into consideration your medical and orthopedic background?*

✓ *Calculated your target heart rate zone?*

✓ *Decided on your fitness goals and matched them with a workout plan using the Exer-Form Chart?*

You're almost there! Now all that remains for you to escape your shape is to:

- Learn the exercises you need to do each time you work out.
- Buy or find access to the equipment you need.
- Follow a workout based on your body type.

## CHAPTER 4

Working Smarter, Not Harder

I'm always dumbfounded by the behavior I see in the health clubs I visit on my travels. On a good day, only one out of ten people starts a workout with a proper warm-up. I'm even more astonished when a client new to Exude who has worked with a personal trainer doesn't know the difference between warming up and stretching. It seems very few people know when or how to stretch. Remember, there is a direct correlation between education and motivation.

Now, you may be thinking, Why is it so important to warm up? To begin with, the benefits are enormous; furthermore, the repercussions of skipping it are serious.

Each and every time you work out, you must do 4 things in the following order: the warm-up, stretching, the workload and the cooldown. There is no negotiating here. If you listen and follow my advice, your chance of injury will be minimized and you will reap the benefits of your fitness regimen. Each phase is as important as the next and together they work synergistically. If you don't perform the phases in this order each time you work out, you will never be truly fit. Nor will you change your body dramatically for the better. We'll start at the beginning.

THE WARM-UP

First off, contrary to belief, warming up is not stretching. And stretching is not warming up. Don't confuse one for the other. Warming up comes before you stretch. The warm-up serves a number of functions:

- It raises your heart rate from its resting state gradually and safely in order to prepare your heart for more demanding activity.
- It provides a smooth transition from the resting state to the higher energy expenditure of the workload phase.
- It prepares the body physiologically and psychologically, decreasing your risk of injury.
- It raises both the general-body and the deep-muscle temperatures and stretches collagenous tissues, which permits greater flexibility.
- It increases your physical working capacity during your workout.

You need to warm up your body the same way you warm up your car before you drive it. Ever try starting your car in cold weather and pulling out of your driveway before the engine warms up? After about 10 feet, the car stalls. Well, the same thing can happen to your body. When you demand too much of it, it can break down. Skipping your warm-up is especially detrimental when you're just starting out on an exercise program. In fact, most heart attacks that occur during exercise or strenuous activities (such as shoveling snow) could be prevented if the victims had only warmed up.

Here's why: warming up gradually raises your heart rate from its resting state. Certain activities (especially anaerobic exercises like lifting a shovelful of heavy snow) *raise* your heart rate quickly—sometimes too quickly—and the stress on the heart can be overwhelming. The result for someone whose heart is not well conditioned could be a heart attack.

Jogging, walking, easy running, stationary biking, swimming, using an aerobic rider, rowing or doing other light aerobic activities are all good ways to warm up. The intensity of this first phase of your workout should *match* your current level of fitness. The more fit you are, the more aggressive you can be with your warm-up. The reason is simple: your heart is in better shape. As your fitness level increases, you can make greater demands on your body.

I'll say it again because it's important: lifting weights is not a warm-up activity. It raises your heart rate too quickly and puts undue stress on your heart. Warm up with *aerobic* activities only.

It takes anywhere from 5 to 15 minutes to warm up. The more fit you are, the less time you need to devote to this part of your workout. You'll know your muscles are warm and your heart ready for more vigorous exercise when you start to break a steady sweat. The colder the weather, the longer you'll need to warm up.

This first phase of your regime should set you up for the rest of your workout. For instance, if you are a long-distance runner, warm up by jogging for 10 minutes or so. The idea is to loosen up the same muscle groups you'll be using later, during your workload.

I've been lecturing you about the importance of warm-up as the start of your body-type workouts, but you should also warm up before engaging in leisure activities as well. Any sport or activity that raises the heart rate considerably—that is, anything that involves quick, concentrated effort—should be preceeded by a warm-up.

I recommend warming up with a stationary bike. It's small, relatively inexpensive and can be easily adjusted so the tension matches your fitness level and body type. It's also far less stressful on your joints and heart than jogging or even walking. At low-tension settings, it raises your heart rate at a slow and a steady pace—something that's especially important for those with heart conditions.

Now you're ready for the second phase of your workout—stretching. Make sure that no more than 5 minutes elapses between warm-up and stretching. If more than 5 minutes pass before you can begin stretching, return to your warm-up activity for a couple of minutes before you stretch.

STRETCHING

Stretching may not be your favorite thing to do. Perhaps you've never been very flexible. Well, I'm happy to report that in my experience advising thousands of clients, everyone—that's right, every man, woman and child—increases their flexibility through stretching. The secret is to warm up first, then stretch major muscle groups in a sequential manner. In other words, you need to perform a series of stretches in a precise order to increase your flexibility and prepare your body for the workload ahead.

To some, flexibility comes easily; to others, it is the most uncomfortable part of working out, but in any event I'm not talking about a big time commitment here. It takes 3 to 5 minutes, depending on your current flexibility. The less flexible you are, the more time you need to devote to stretching. The more flexible you are, the less you need to stretch. As you age, you need to spend a little more time stretching. If you have tight hamstrings but flexible quadriceps, spend a little more time stretching your hamstrings as well as anywhere else you feel tight.

As an added benefit, stretching increases your range of motion, which allows your muscles to grow and respond faster. Golfers and tennis players, hear this: you can add 20 yards to your drive or 15 to 30 miles per hour to your serve by simply increasing your range of motion. In fact, you can take all the golf and tennis lessons in the world but if you have poor flexibility, it will be hard to improve the length of your drive or the speed of your serve. In fact, you can enhance your performance in any sport by modestly improving your flexibility.

Have you noticed people at your gym who have worked hard and diligently for years with no visible improvements? Part of the reason their bodies don't shape up is because they don't stretch. It's especially important if you're trying to firm up your body. If you took two people of the same age, height, weight and genetic makeup and body type and instructed just one to include stretching in their workout, the one who stretched would have better body tone and overall fitness. I know this to be true, and not just because I've read studies about it in every major medical journal. I've seen it in the bodies of many frustrated and unhappy regular exercisers out there. They sweat and sweat, thinking and hoping that one day their bodies will change for the better, but they don't.

Genetics do play a role in flexibility, but everyone can increase flexibility with the proper techniques. I know plenty of athletes as strong as oxen who are constantly pulling muscles, particularly their hamstrings. This is usually due to overtraining and lack of flexibility. Certain exercises either increase or decrease your flexibility. For example, jogging and running tend to tighten your hamstrings; biking tightens the quadriceps (the front of your thigh); and weight lifting—especially power lifting—can tighten the entire body but wreaks havoc with the shoulder and back regions. Stretching doesn't make you immune to injury, but if you stretch, you'll minimize your risk and the severity of injury.

Good flexibility increases your resistance to injury by definition. *Being flexible* means you have a wide range of movement within your joints, so ligaments and other collagenous tissues are not so easily strained or torn. Conversely, hyperflexibility must be avoided, because loose-jointed individuals are more prone to dislocations and other injuries. Extremes in flexibility are of little value and can ultimately weaken joints. Like strength, flexibility is specific to the joint and its surrounding complementary tissues.

The correct way to stretch is with relaxed, sustained poses

known as static stretching. Don't bounce up and down (called ballistic stretching) or stretch until you feel pain, which can do more harm than good.

Stretch until you feel a mild tension, and relax as you hold the stretch for 30 to 60 seconds. The feeling of tension should subside slightly. If it does not, ease off a bit and find a degree of tension that is comfortable. As your flexibility improves, try stretching slightly farther. Again the tension should lessen as you hold the stretch; if not, ease off slightly.

Breathe normally, exhaling as you bend forward and then in and out as you hold your stretch. Do not hold your breath and do try to relax your facial muscles. If a stretch position prohibits normal breathing, then you are obviously not relaxed. Ease up on the stretch until you can breathe comfortably. In the beginning, silently count to 30 for each stretch. As you become more practiced, you won't need to count. You'll know your muscles are loose by the way they feel.

Remember, stretching takes place only *after* the warm-up phase. For those who are very inflexible, I recommend yoga. Yoga by itself, however, is not the path to true fitness. Flexibility is just one component of the fitness equation.

THE WORKLOAD

The workload portion of your fitness routine must be well organized and orchestrated *before* you start exercising. You'll be working at the highest intensity during your workload, with your muscles warm and loose from the first 2 parts of your workout. In fact, you cannot effectively train at a high intensity unless you have warmed up and stretched.

Your workload is the "meat" of your fitness regimen, determined by your goals. If you have allotted an hour and 15 minutes toward your workout, your time might break down like this: 10 minutes warm-up; 5 minutes stretching; 55 minutes workload; and 5 minutes cooldown.

What you choose to do during those 55 workload minutes should be governed by the following:

- your goals (weight loss or toning)
- your body type (which will dictate the kinds of exercises you should be performing)
- your orthopedic and medical background (which dictate which exercises you should avoid)
- your present level of fitness (which determines the intensity of your efforts)

There's a lot to consider, and that's why it's imperative to plan your routine *before* you start exercising.

With the proper planning, you can smoothly transition from stretching to the workload phase. Your medley of exercises needs to be choreographed like a ballet. No talking, no gossiping! You're focused, blocking out all negative thoughts and worries. You may speak to others while you're warming up or stretching, but during your workload, you need to be completely absorbed in what you're doing, shielded from outside stressors.

If you work out at a gym or a health club, take a look around the next time you're there and note what you see. If it's like 99 percent of the gyms I've visited, most of the people are talking, laughing or watching somebody else—not engrossed in their own workout. And who could blame them? Working out at a health club today has become more of a fashion show than a focused commitment to fitness. Even I find it hard to concentrate on exercising in a club environment.

Here's an interesting tidbit: of all the people who have come into Exude for advice on exercise, the people who work out at home are more fit, better informed, more focused and more consistent than those who work out exclusively at gyms. The at-home exercisers were also more apt to exercise while traveling than the clubbies. Why? Well, people who train at home usually do not have as much discretionary time as those who work out at a club or gym. They're people who have integrated their workout plan realistically into their lives—better, in fact, than other exercisers do. They are also more self-motivated and they make adjustments to consistently make time for exercise.

The average workload phase is about 50 minutes, which you can split up any number of ways. Let's say you're moderately fit and your goal is to lose, say, 20 pounds. The Exer-Form Chart (page 68) will provide you with the correct percent of aerobic vs. anaerobic exercise. In this case you'll be doing quite a bit of moderately intense aerobic exercise with some anaerobic work blended in.

How do you decide what to do when? Well, I've created detailed beginner, active, and very active workouts to eliminate the guesswork (Part Two), but when I create individualized regimes for my clients, I always suggest that after a cardio interval, they start out with the exercise they dislike the most.

Let's say abs are your least favorite exercise. Your workload routine might look something like this: 15 minutes jumping rope, 5 minutes riding a stationary bike, 15 minutes doing abdominal, leg and hip exercises, 10 minutes doing upper-body exercises with a weight bar and 5 minutes jumping rope.

If you wait until the end of your routine to do the thing you most dread, chances are you won't do it, so avoid self-sabotage by tackling those abs, for example, immediately.

Increasing Intensity

Learning how and when to increase the intensity of your workload will take some time to master. Some people don't know where to begin. Take Michael, for instance. I met this 40-year-old businessman in a social setting through some mutual friends. When he learned I was a fitness expert, he asked me for some advice. He explained that a couple of years before, he had decided to lose some weight and get in shape. Aside from high school sports, he'd never really exercised regularly, so he joined a local health club. Two years later, he hasn't really seen that much change and he wondered what he might be doing wrong.

Let's see if you can figure it out. He goes to the gym 3 or 4 times a week and spends about an hour there on each visit. He walks for 30 to 45 minutes, stretches, and exercises his upper body with free weights. Sounds good so far, doesn't it? I ask Michael how fast he walks, and if he ever jogs. He says he sets the treadmill speed at 3.2 miles per hour.

Are you getting the picture? I look at him and think to myself, Why can't this 40-year-old, 160-pound man who is in relatively good health walk any faster than 3.2 miles an hour? I look him in the eye and ask how fast he was walking when he started out two years ago.

I can tell he sees the light when he sheepishly answers, "Three-point-two miles an hour."

Don't get me wrong. It's absolutely great that he goes to the gym regularly, but working out should involve work! It's okay to be slightly out of breath, and yes, you're supposed to break a sweat. Going for a leisurely walk after dinner is good for you, but it's not exercise per se. If you want to burn fat and calories and improve your cardiovascular health, you need to work out with the proper intensity right from the beginning. You need to elevate your heart rate and maintain it in your training zone.

Other folks have a difficult time distinguishing intensity from pain. Say you're jumping rope for 2 minutes and you're out of breath. At first you may equate being out of breath with fatigue. You think you can't go on. Perhaps it's because you've never experienced this feeling before, or perhaps you fear injuring yourself. Whatever the reason, you've got to push through those feelings because the bottom line is that you must increase your intensity in order to reach your goals.

Instead of stopping and giving up, get on the stationary bike or walk around for a minute or 2. Let your heart rate come down a bit, then go right back to it. Picking up that jump rope for another minute or so will raise your cardiovascular conditioning. You can do it, and do it safely by staying in tune with your body. Don't be too hard on yourself, though. The first few times you follow an escape-your-shape workout may be a real challenge. You'll feel very different than 2, 3 and 4 months down the line.

As you become physically and psychologically accustomed to your new workout regime, you'll find that you can easily perform your workload because you're getting fitter and fitter. You'll take a certain pride in the fact that you've mastered the exercises, but you should also recognize that feeling as an indicator that you're ready to take it to the next level. There's no doubt about it, ramping things up takes mental toughness, but it's worth it.

How do you do it? Well, the workouts in Part Two are designed for beginners, active, and very active exercisers. Jumping from the beginner to the active workout, or from active to very active is one way to ramp up. But you'll also want to do some fine-tuning. To learn more about how to intensify your workout appropriately for your body type, look for the intensity headings in the workout chapters in Part Two.

FOR BEGINNERS AND THOSE WHO ARE MODERATELY FIT, increase the duration of all aerobic activities as well as the number of repetitions for all anaerobic exercises. That means, for example, increasing the time you jump rope from 3 to 4 to 5 minutes and beyond and lifting that weight bar over your head another 5, then 10 times.

FOR THOSE CONFIDENT ABOUT THEIR ADVANCED FITNESS LEVEL, increase the resistance, tension or incline on aerobic equipment (when body type allows) and/or add more weight for all anaerobic exercises. In other words, if you can jog easily for 20 minutes on a treadmill with no incline, try jogging the same length of time on a 2 or 3 percent grade; if you have no trouble curling a 4-pound weight bar 50 times, try using an 8-pound bar the next time.

It's important to put some thought into how you're going to increase the intensity of your workload without adding many minutes to your aerobic intervals and additional sets to your exercises. If you're like most of my clients, you can't afford to increase the time you devote to exercise. If keeping to your regime means having to find more time, you might not stick to it.

Contrary to popular belief, you do not need to dramatically alter your routine or buy expensive new pieces of equipment to keep improving the way your body looks. You can keep things simple and increase your intensity using the same fitness equipment you begin with, though you may ultimately use it a little differently. You'll add new exercises when you've outgrown old ones. You'll drop exercises which are no longer as effective as they once were. If you don't, you'll be exercising for hours on end, and no one has time for that.

So, whether you take exercise classes, lift weights, work out on weight machines, run, swim, row or practice any other form of exercise, you need to keep increasing intensity until you've met the following criteria:

1. Your fitness program is well balanced—you have nice flexibility, muscle strength, muscle endurance, cardiovascular efficiency and a good body ratio of lean body mass vs. fat.
2. If you're involved in a sport, you can participate at a level that you're completely satisfied with.
3. You're at the weight and body-fat percent that you are happy with.
4. You've met all of your health goals—blood pressure, cholesterol level, resting heart rate.
5. You fit comfortably in your clothes.
6. You look and feel great!

Increasing your exercise intensity is a skill, a skill that can be learned with patience and practice. I emphasize patience because too often, people who come to see me at Exude have wildly unrealistic goals. They want to be fit in a week! Others want to lose 10 pounds in 2 weeks. I could go on and on, but the point here is that when you're too aggressive with your fitness regimen, you're bound to injure yourself. Remember, if you injure yourself while exercising, you cannot be consistent. And if you're not consistent, you'll never reach your weight-loss or any other goals.

To recap:

- In order to raise your fitness level and change your body, you need to increase your intensity.
- When you can perform a given exercise with ease, that's an indication that you should ramp up your intensity.
- If you're just starting out or are moderately fit, increase your intensity by extending the duration of your chosen exercise and/or the number of repetitions; if you're confident about your fitness level, increase resistance and weight.
- At some point, you'll need to discard exercises you've mastered and replace them with more challenging ones.

I like to tell my clients that learning how to exercise properly is like taking a course in college. If you attend all the classes and keep up with your homework, at exam time you will be prepared.

The same holds true for your fitness routine; educate yourself on the best exercise suited for you and be consistent and the rest will take care of itself. In my twenty years in the fitness business, I have never worked with anyone who exercised properly and consistently who did not change his or her body for the better—not one! Everyone can escape their shape and improve how they look through proper fitness. By the end of this book, you will be able to identify what, if any, changes that you would like or need to make in your fitness regimen.

Now all that's left is the fourth and final phase of your workout—the cooldown.

THE COOLDOWN

The cooldown is the shortest of all the phases of your workout, 3 to 5 minutes, depending upon the intensity of your workout. The cooldown takes only a couple of minutes to complete, but the minutes are essential, so don't neglect them, or the repercussions of skipping them can be severe. The purpose of this phase of your workout is to gradually slow your heart rate and a myriad of other body functions to pre-exercise levels. By cooling down, your body is able to adapt to the shock that you just put it through. Specifically, the blood and muscle lactic acid levels decrease swiftly during your cooldown. I recommend mild aerobic exercises at this time—stationary biking (with little or no tension), walking (with no incline), slow jogging, swimming leisurely, rowing (with no resistance) and using an aerobic rider. Do *not* cool down with anaerobic exercises, which do not gradually lower your heart rate.

I don't recommend stretching as a cool down. If you want to stretch after your workout, cool down first and then stretch. Be careful here, though. Certain muscles might be fatigued from your workout and are more susceptible to being strained or pulled. And because stretching raises your heart rate from its current state, it is not as safe or effective for gradually bringing your heart rate down from your THR.

Here's another way of looking at the cooldown process: You start your workout by warming up, gradually increasing your heart rate. During your workload your heart rate rises considerably and for an extended period of time. In order to bring your heart rate back down toward your pre-exercise level, you need to keep moving your body but gradually decrease the intensity of your activity. How long you should cool down is dictated by the length and intensity of your workout, but, as I said, anywhere from 3 to 5 minutes should be sufficient. If you feel you need more time, then take a few extra minutes. Your breathing should return to normal and your pulse should return to under a 100 beats per minute within a few minutes of finishing your workload phase.

By properly and sufficiently cooling down, you also greatly decrease the chances of cardiac complications associated with a wide array of heart conditions.

YOUR FITNESS TOOLS—WHAT YOU NEED

Over the years, I've seen thousands of people who travel, work long hours and don't have a lot of time or money to devote to fitness. Although they had lifestyle constraints, I knew that I could find solutions for them. And there are solutions that can help you exercise properly and consistently, too. My clients' lifestyle and other constraints helped me to mold my fitness programs, which can be performed anywhere. I focused on developing a fitness system that would work for all ages, shapes, levels of fitness and, most important, could work in the home if one couldn't afford or make time to get to the gym.

As a result, the fitness equipment you'll need in order to follow the workouts in Part Two is inexpensive, effective and space efficient. Living in New York City, where personal space is limited and expensive, influenced this program also. In fact, you need only 6 square feet of space to complete any of the body-type workouts and you can choose to work out inside or in the great outdoors. Even those of you who have turned making excuses into a fine art can't hide anymore. You can do these workouts anywhere—on the road, in your living room, or in a park. Listed below is the fitness equipment you'll need to perform the prescribed workouts. The only piece of fitness equipment that you may substitute is the aerobic piece; be sure that whatever you use, the activity is conducive to your body type. The good news is that you'll never need to add pieces of fitness apparatus, even as you progress. What will change, however, is how you use the pieces you have as you become more fit and your body starts to improve.

Every body-type workout utilizes the following fitness equipment:

1. ONE PIECE OF AEROBIC EQUIPMENT, PREFERABLY A STATIONARY BIKE, EITHER UPRIGHT OR RECUMBENT. RATIONALE: Stationary bikes are small, inexpensive, adjustable regarding the resistance and tension based on your body type and current level of fitness and are appropriate for *all* body types. If you have certain medical or orthopedic constraints and cannot jump rope, you can still interval train (alternate biking with other activities) without putting undue stress on your back, hips and feet. See the Body Type and Aerobic Fitness Equipment Chart on p. 50 for additional information on your body type.

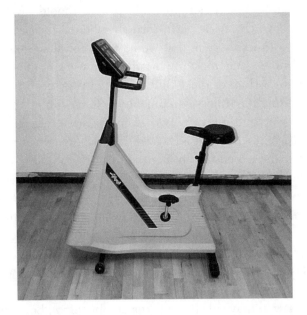

2. A JUMP ROPE. RATIONALE: It's simply the best piece of fitness equipment ever invented. It's cheap, takes up virtually no room in your closet or suitcase and provides great aerobic exercise for every body type. Need I say more? Okay, it burns more calories per minute than almost any other form of aerobic exercise and is the only known piece of fitness equipment that helps eliminate cellulite. Jumping rope works both upper and lower bodies and can help improve your performance in any sport.

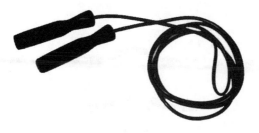

3. A FIRM EXERCISE MAT OR DUAL-IMPACT MAT. RATIONALE: It's important to perform your abdominals and other calisthenics on a surface that is firm yet giving enough to support your back. Every body-type workout includes abdominal exercises. A dual-impact mat can do double duty with abdominal exercises and as a forgiving surface for those who do not have wooden floors at home to jump rope on.

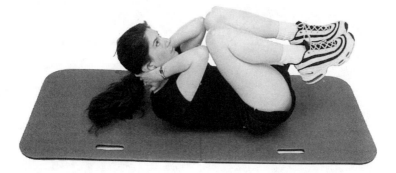

4. A FOLDING 4-POUND AEROBIC BAR. RATIONALE: This light, portable bar is a part of every body-type workout. It's great for stretching, upper-body exercises, lower-body calisthenics and side benders and is integral for toning and reducing hips, thighs and abs. For Hourglasses, Cones, overweight Rulers and overweight Spoons, this bar is also used for all upper-body exercises.

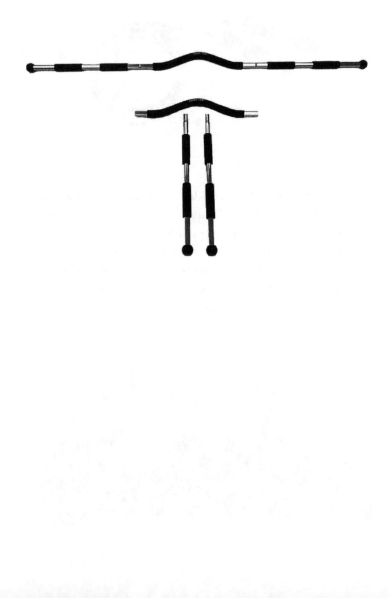

5. A 10-, 15- OR 20-POUND CURL OR STRAIGHT BAR. RATIONALE:
It's important for both men and women to perform upper-body
exercises with resistance in order to tone, build muscle and
combat osteoporosis. I recommend a higher weight for men, 15
or 20 pounds. For women, 10 pounds is plenty. Women who
need to lose weight and mass should start with the 4-pound
aerobic bar and perform lots of repetitions. All of the bars are
small, easy to carry and can also be used for a variety of leg-
strengthening exercises.

There you have it, all the fitness equipment you'll ever need.
Remember, *don't substitute* any of the above except for your
aerobic piece, and then only if it is recommended for your body
type.

Now you can choose your body-type workout and start
moving!

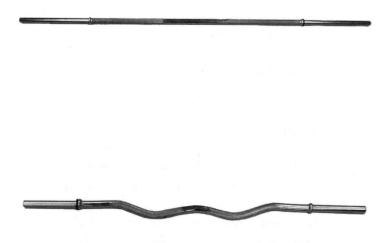

CHAPTER 5

The Jump Rope,
Your Secret Weapon

I've included this section on jumping rope because it is by far the most effective and efficient aerobic exercise, one that I recommend everybody incorporate into the aerobic portion of their workload. That means you'll need to warm up and stretch before you jump.

Before I get into the how-to, let me begin with a few words of encouragement. I often see looks of dismay from clients when I first introduce this activity into their fitness prescription, and I understand why. Many who come to me for guidance (and perhaps you, too) harbor misconceptions about the difficulty or the strain that jumping rope puts on your body. Let me lay some of those worries to rest.

Fact or Fallacy?
FALLACY: Jumping rope is high impact.

FACT: Not so. Actually it is lower impact than jogging or running.

FALLACY: Jumping rope is bad for your knees.

FACT: Actually, when done properly, it can strengthen the tissues that surround and support the knees and ankles.

FALLACY: Jumping rope is bad for your back.

FACT: Jumping rope can help strengthen your back. **But don't dive into a jump rope routine if** you are suffering from any pain or discomfort to your back or any other part of your body. Consult your health care professional first.

FALLACY: Jumping rope is too hard to learn and difficult to do and requires a lot of coordination.

FACT: Jumping rope is easy to learn, no matter how uncoordinated you think you are. What's hard is building up endurance, something that requires commitment and mental toughness as much as physical ability. The key is patience and building your stamina slowly.

FALLACY: Jumping rope is for kids.

FACT: We may have started jumping rope in the schoolyard, but you can jump rope at any age. Athletes use jump ropes to stay fit and improve their sports performance, coordination, stamina and agility.

FALLACY: You need to be in great shape before you can start jumping rope.

FACT: Actually, you can begin jumping rope no matter what your fitness level. You might start off with just 10, 20 or even 30 jumps, but you will progress quickly as your fitness level improves.

Jumping rope is the only exercise that streamlines your entire body. That's right, it's for anyone trying to shed excess weight or mass. I've seen thousands of clients over the past 20 years incorporate jumping rope into their workouts with amazing results. Remember that no one picks up a rope and jumps for 5 minutes straight right off the bat. It will take time to build your endurance, but you can do it. I've seen it myself with clients who could barely complete 10 revolutions to begin with; today they can keep it up for 30 minutes at a stretch!

WHAT'S SO GREAT ABOUT JUMPING ROPE?

Jumping rope will burn a substantial amount of calories in a relatively short period of time—more than 23 calories per minute! Compare that to stationary biking at 10 MPH, which burns only 6 calories per minute, or brisk walking (4 MPH), which burns only 7 calories per minute. If your fitness goals include losing weight, be sure to include jumping rope in your off-day routine.

Jumping rope burns fat throughout your entire body and works both your upper and lower bodies simultaneously. The result is that you'll have better muscle tone and definition all over. In addition, it has a positive effect on your performance in whatever sports or activities you enjoy. Specifically you'll be able to move faster and with better coordination, balance and agility. Need I say more? Okay, jumping rope frees you from expensive equipment, gyms and trainers. And it's totally portable so you can work out just about anywhere.

Whether you jump rope alone or in a class, it's always challenging. You'll never become bored or outgrow it. It's fun and, best of all, incredibly motivating because you'll see noticeable improvement in the way you look and feel right from the start. I never feel more energized, accomplished or fit than when I finish a jump rope routine. Once you start, you won't want to stop, either!

THE BENEFITS OF JUMPING ROPE

Is one of the highest fat-burning aerobic activities

Burns fat throughout your body

Produces visible results in a short period of time

Improves cardiovascular health and aerobic capacity

Helps reduce cellulite

Strengthens, tones and defines all major muscles in the upper and lower bodies

Improves coordination, balance, stamina and agility

Is completely portable, great for traveling

BEFORE YOU START

Start off on the right foot by properly equipping yourself with the following:

A JUMP ROPE. You'll want to start out with a speed rope. When you need to increase the intensity of your workload, you may advance to a peg rope, unless it's contraindicated for your body type. Avoid cloth ropes, which don't have the same heft. They tend to tangle and their lighter weight means you just can't build the same momentum.

A word about length: To be sure your jump rope is the correct length for you, grip the rope by the handles, hold the center of the rope to the floor with one foot, and pull the handles up toward your shoulders. The ends of the handles should just about reach your armpits (see photo 1). If you need to shorten the

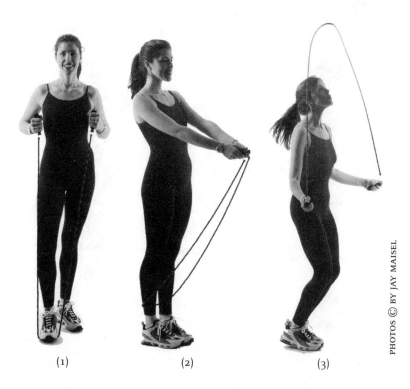

(1)   (2)   (3)

PHOTOS © BY JAY MAISEL

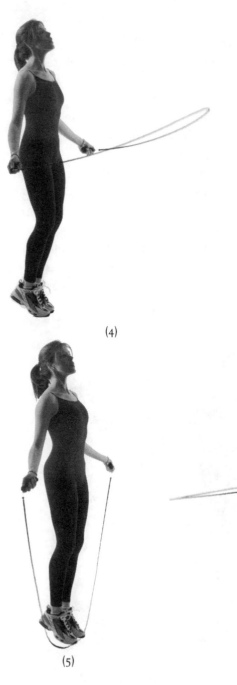

NOTE: You will need to exaggerate the forward, circular motion of your forearms (perhaps you'll even need to use your upper arms and shoulders) to begin the rotation of the rope. Thereafter, the motion becomes more compact and abbreviated.

(4)

(5)

(6)

PHOTOS © BY JAY MAISEL

rope, you can tie a knot in the rope near the point where the rope meets the handle. Don't tie knots in the center of the rope—they'll only trip you up.

CROSS TRAINERS. While jumping rope isn't as high impact as running or jogging, you still need a pair of good shoes that will cushion the balls of your feet. Don't forget socks!

A FORGIVING SURFACE. Make sure to jump on a surface that gives, like wood floors with a good subflooring, a dual-impact mat, or short grass.

WATER. Keep a bottle on hand so you can take small sips throughout your workout. You'll sweat a lot, and you don't want to dehydrate.

BASIC JUMP

With the correct grip (see the illustration on the following page), hold the handles out in front of you with the rope behind you draped below the calves (see photo 2). Keeping your feet together, your hands move down and to your sides. As you rotate your forearms forward, down and around in a circular motion, the rope comes up behind you and over your head (see photos 3–6). As the rope moves toward the floor in front of you (it should strike the floor between 6 to 12 inches in front of your feet), jump about 1 inch while you maintain the circular motion of your forearms. Then, as the rope passes under your feet, gently land on the balls of your feet. It is the continuous circular movement of your forearms that keeps the rope moving down under your feet and then up over your head again and again.

Your palms should be facing slightly upward, your elbows should be 3 to 6 inches from your sides, and your hands should be slightly in front of you, about level with your hips. Keep your hands moving continuously in compact forward circular motions, so that the rope keeps turning. Don't worry or give up if you can jump only a few times before you miss. Nobody picks

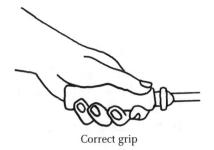

Correct grip

up a rope and jumps perfectly right off the bat! When you miss, just start again. Remember, it is the number of cumulative jumps that count. A few jumps will turn into 10, then 20, and soon you'll start counting minutes.

INCREASING INTENSITY

With time you'll master the goals you first set out for yourself both physically and psychologically.

DURATION. When you can easily turn that rope 100 times, you should increase the duration of your routine, but do it gradually. Try jumping 125, then 150, then 200 revolutions before you start counting minutes.

FOOTWORK. Practicing different footwork is another way to increase the intensity of your jump rope intervals and works other muscles in your legs. Try the following step variations for 20 jumps, returning to the basic jump for 20 jumps in between. As you master each of these, you'll want to increase the number of jumps for each in intervals of 5 (25, 30, 40, up to 100):

1. Shift your weight to one foot and then the other—as you become comfortable with this pattern, it may become your basic jump. That is, you'll return to it between intervals of other footwork.
2. Run in place.
3. Alternate jumping with your feet spread apart and then together (as you would do a jumping jack).

4. Alternate kicking one leg out to the side, then the other.
5. Lift one knee, then the other.
6. Jump with your feet together from side to side, as if you're skiing and making quick sharp turns.

If you become fatigued or short of breath, don't stop moving. Instead, switch to active-rest moves such as side benders. When you catch your breath, pick up the rope again.

TROUBLESHOOTING

If you are having trouble with jumping rope, check yourself against the following guidelines:

- Keep your hands at your sides, just slightly in front of your hips at waist height.
- Stand up straight with knees slightly bent. Don't hunch your shoulders or bend over at the waist.
- Don't look down at your feet or lower your head.
- Don't snap your wrists—move your forearms, wrists and hands as a unit. Keep the wrists firm but flexible. Don't overrotate or swivel your hands.
- Practice in front of a mirror if you are having trouble on a particular move.
- If you find yourself double jumping (jumping twice for each revolution of the rope), slow down. Practice jumping at a slower, steady speed before you pick up the pace.
- Jump so that your feet come off the surface no more than an inch or so.
- Establish a rhythm and coordinate the pace of your feet with your hands. Let your hands lead, and your feet will follow.

For more information on jumping rope, log on to www.exude.com, and click onto "Jumping Towards Fitness".

CHAPTER 6

Exercise and Diet, the Dynamic Weight-Loss Duo

Weight loss can be achieved *only* by creating a caloric deficit. This caloric deficit can be done in a number of ways: with proper and consistent exercise, with a reduction of your caloric intake, or with a combination of the 2. The best way to lose weight and keep it off is to do a combination. There is no other healthy way to lose weight permanently. In fact, in my 20 years in the fitness business, I have never met anyone who has reached their weight, aesthetic and fitness goals through diet alone—not one! I have seen people struggle for years with all kinds of diets. Some lose weight and drop a size but often they actually look *fatter* than the scale indicates because their ratio of lean muscle to body fat is so poor. Thus, they don't look much different at all.

Take, for example, Melissa, a Spoon, who is 5'4" and weighs 140 pounds. She decides to "go on a diet" and loses 10 pounds. When she weighs 130 pounds, she doesn't look that different. In fact, her problem areas—her hips, thighs and buttocks—look the same. Here's why: when you lose weight by dieting alone, your body's ability to burn fat slows down considerably because your Basic Metabolic Rate (BMR) decreases. And many—especially those who do not have a healthy body ratio to begin with—

can actually lose weight while simultaneously increasing their body-fat percentage. Melissa may have lost weight, but was that really her goal? Didn't she also expect to drop a dress size or look better proportioned? Focusing on scale weight can actually hinder your efforts to tone and trim your body.

I have seen countless clients follow my escape-your-shape routine without changing their diet at all and lose from 12 to 20 inches off their bodies! That's right, their scales showed no weight loss, but what a difference in their appearance! Remember, this can be achieved only through consistent exercise based on your body type. More than 20,000 clients have shown me that proper exercise can work wonders, but you cannot dramatically improve your body and escape your shape by dieting alone.

Similar to exercising, eating properly requires commitment. Sometimes it takes years before good eating habits become an ingrained part of our behavior. It's not easy. I have met with hundreds of individuals who want to lose weight and decide to "diet" first. They think they'll lose the weight before engaging in a fitness program. Guess what? Chances are, they'll never get to the exercise part of the plan. The reason is that when they go on a low-calorie diet, they have less fuel and as a result don't have the energy to exercise at all. Sure, they can walk or slow jog for a ½ hour or so, but that won't burn many calories. They may well lose weight, but will lack good muscle tone.

On the other hand, I have seen clients so energized by a new fitness program and the positive changes it produces that they're eager to see what additional benefits they can reap from better eating habits. The result is a person who exercises, eats well, loses weight and improves the overall look and feel of their body.

There is synergy there. The two can work dramatic changes together. Eating and exercising properly is the goal, but rarely can people master both from the outset. That's why I always say a great exercise program can make up for a poor diet, but a great diet can never make up for lack of exercise!

WHAT YOU NEED TO KNOW ABOUT YOUR DIET

My belief is that no one should be totally restrictive when it comes to eating. I myself strive for balance, and it is this balance we teach our clients as well. Nine times out of ten deprivation leads to failure, and let's face it, that isn't much fun, either. Life involves eating. I would be lying to you if I said that I don't enjoy a beer or a glass of wine with my dinner a few nights a week, or that I do not indulge in an occasional sweet. I also do not endorse any fad diets such as low-carb, high-protein or no-fat or no-carb diet plans. The only reason any of these diets are popular is that we as a nation (and I know we're not alone) do not have enough self-control when it comes to portion size. As children we ate pasta and meatballs, salad and a sensible dessert and somehow never gained weight. Why? I'll tell you. First we were given controlled amounts of food. We also ate balanced meals and didn't lounge around after eating; we played hide-and-seek or cowboys and Indians. In other words, we *moved* . . . a lot more than most of us do now. We did not go on fad diets. We did not eliminate entire food groups.

While fad diets work for some people initially, the human body was simply not designed to eat steak 7 days a week. Our bodies still require a balance of carbs, protein and fats in order to function our best both mentally and physically.

Your lifestyle dictates where and when you eat just as it determines where and when you exercise. It does not, however, dictate the amount you choose to eat or the type of food you eat, either. We must learn how to eat properly when we're on the road or at a restaurant.

I live by one rule of thumb when it comes to eating and maintaining my ideal weight: On the days I exercise, I know I can afford to eat a *little* more. On the days that I do not work out, I try to lower my caloric intake. And if I fail to limit my calorie intake on the days that I am not exercising (it happens to all of us sometimes), I make sure that the next day I work out a little longer to make up for the extra calories consumed the day before. It's all about balance. I rarely overindulge and then sit around for days without exercising because I would certainly start to gain weight. You cannot allow more than a day or two to go by without exercising and expect to gain no weight if you are taking in more calories than you are expending. Those who are trying to lose a few pounds or maintain their weight can get away with it occasionally. But for most of you who are trying to lose weight, what you eat and how much you exercise should be bonded inseparably in your mind.

DIET TYPES

To attain your weight-loss goals, you must first *accept* the fact that you can't take off those unwanted pounds, much less keep them off, without proper and regular exercise. But don't despair, once you come to terms with this, you can explore options that fit your lifestyle and motivation level. You can lose weight without starving yourself or knocking yourself out mentally and physically at the gym.

When you're trying to lose weight, it's important to understand yourself and, more important, embrace what you *actually* do rather than what you *think* you're going to do. In order to lose weight, you need a plan that includes a doable exercise routine and reasonable limitations on what you eat. Are you really ready to embrace both? If not, make an honest self-assessment. Some of you love to exercise while others hate it. Some love to eat; others have little trouble saying no to seconds or dessert. Listed below are 4 diet types I have identified based on behavior patterns I've observed in my clients. Each type is characterized by the amount of exercise they're willing to do versus their willingness to change their eating patterns in order to lose weight. Which type best describes you?

RATIONAL INDIVIDUAL. You are someone who enjoys and chooses to exercise 4 or 5 days per week on a consistent basis and you're willing to make small dietary changes in order to see weight loss.

ACCEPTING INDIVIDUAL. You are willing to work out 2 or 3 days per week, but do it only because you know it is good for you, and you watch carefully what you eat on a day-to-day basis so that you can lose weight.

EXCESSIVE INDIVIDUAL. You are willing to work out 6 or even 7 days per week, but you want no boundaries when it comes to watching what you eat. You rely solely on exercise for weight loss.

CONTENTIOUS INDIVIDUAL. You loathe exercise and are willing to exercise only 1, maybe 2 days per week, but will follow a strict diet and watch every little morsel you put in your mouth. You rely on "diet" 90 percent to achieve your weight-loss goals.

These types represent the entire spectrum of weight-loss behaviors. Ideally, you want to imitate the behavior of the first type—the rational individual. A combination of exercising and sensibly restricting caloric intake is the most effective way to lose weight, but the reality of the situation is that you may never be willing or able to exercise 4 or 5 days per week, and that's okay. However, you can't exercise one or two days per week, eat excessively and expect to lose weight. You can't even maintain your current weight with that plan. In fact, you'll most certainly gain. Accept your personality type and make the best of it. The reason I implore you to exercise with more frequency and to try to make small dietary changes is because over the long haul, it is the least stressful approach, and the one you are more apt to stick with.

THE NUMBERS GAME

I'm always fascinated and bewildered at the response I get when I suggest a plan to a new client that will yield them a loss of 1 pound per week. It goes something like this:

"Oh, Edward, that's not enough, I want to lose three or four pounds per week."

"Tell me, Karen," I ask, "how long have you been twenty pounds overweight?"

"For about twelve years."

"Let me get this straight. For twelve years you have *accepted* yourself being twenty pounds overweight and I'm telling you that in twenty weeks you can be at a healthy and fit weight, and that's not good enough?"

Karen assures me that she's willing to do everything and anything I ask in order to speed up the process. The only trouble is that "everything" can't include extra workouts ("I have a really hectic job and I travel a lot.") or changes to her diet ("I'm a vegetarian so I'm already eating well!").

That's when I explain "calories in = calories out." That phrase describes the situation in which the total number of calories that you consume on a particular day is the same amount of calories you burn during that same stretch of time. And when that happens, you will neither lose nor gain weight, but rather break even. Your weight will remain the same. When your caloric intake *exceeds* the number of calories you are burning, you gain weight, and unless you do something to change that situation, you'll continue to gain. When you create a deficit (burn more calories than you consume), you lose weight. Understanding the formula is the easy part. The real challenge is to maintain a deficit until you reach your goals. And by the way, I don't care how well you think you eat, if you take in more calories than you expend, it doesn't matter if you are eating carrots or Snickers bars, you will gain weight. Your body doesn't discriminate when it comes to calories. It doesn't matter where they come from. Sure, if you eat carrots, you'll be healthier, but not thinner.

Then comes my favorite part. I follow up with clients like Karen, who claim to be willing to do "anything," by asking whether they're planning to move, change jobs or their everyday routine in order to help them meet their deadline. Of course they're not. I'm quick to enlighten them that the odds of their exercising more than 3 or 4 times per week given their other commitments are not good. In addition, due to the travel and stress they endure, it will take some time after establishing the food adjustments necessary to achieve their weight-loss goals. After a few minutes, most recognize that there's a gap between what they want and what they're willing to do to get it. The truth is, losing 1 pound per week, week after week is a tremendous achievement.

Remember, it's not just a pound of weight that falls away, but inches as well. No scale can measure that. Say after the first week on your new program you weigh yourself and the scale hasn't budged, though you feel thinner and your clothes feel looser. Are you going to let the fact that you didn't "lose weight" that week set a negative tone that may last for days? That's why I tell everyone to take measurements, because for *some* people, it's not weight they need to lose as much as fat and inches. In fact, I recommend that unless you have more than 15 pounds to lose, you weigh yourself no more than once a month. For those who need to lose more than 15 pounds, no more than once a week. Use scale weight as a checkpoint, but don't beat yourself up over what the scale says. Whether you lose weight, remain the same or gain weight during that time period, you can reflect back on your behavior and make whatever adjustments might be necessary. Maybe you worked out often but did not watch what you ate, or maybe you carefully watched your food intake but worked out very little or not at all. Perhaps you simply need to ramp up your intensity. Whatever the weight loss or gain, there is always a behavioral reason behind it.

Be patient with yourself. Just as it takes time to develop "bad" habits—like not exercising properly or consistently, or eating too much—it takes time to make proper exercise a consistent part of your life and to adjust your food intake to match your lifestyle. I suggest working toward intermediate goals. For example, when you're consistently completing 3 body-type workouts a week, try to exercise 4 or 5 days in a row (with the off-day routines on the fourth and/or fifth days), or try to make some subtle changes to your diet, like eliminating desserts or limiting alcohol consumption. Make a small change each week. Try working out a little longer or maybe with a bit more intensity. Putting it all together takes time and perseverance. That's why I tell people like Karen not to focus too much on weight loss. The *real* goal is to create a clear path to exercising and eating properly and consistently. That way, the weight you lose will stay off forever.

HOW MUCH IS ENOUGH?

How much is another common blunder I encounter with those just starting out on a fitness program, especially the millions of people who walk for fitness—and who do only that for exercise. They think that because they are "working out," they can eat whatever they want. Sure, you walk for a half hour or even a full hour daily, but you are burning only 200 to 400 calories during that process. Because you exercised that day, you felt that you could eat more, so proceeded to have a drink or two before dinner, an appetizer, a complete dinner and, to "reward" yourself for that invigorating walk, a great-tasting dessert. Unfortunately, you just inhaled 1000 more calories than you expended on that particular day. At this pace, you'll gain 2 pounds a week (3500 calories equals 1 pound), without even batting an eye. To maintain your current weight, calories in must equal calories out, remember?

How many calories should you consume daily? I have found the following formula very helpful in determining the amount of calories you should consume on a day-to-day basis in order to lose weight*:

---

* PLEASE NOTE: THIS FORMULA IS JUST AN AVERAGE AND MAY OR MAY NOT BE AN ACCURATE GUIDE TO YOUR CALORIC NEEDS. FOR A CUSTOMIZED ASSESSMENT OF YOUR CALORIC AND NUTRITIONAL NEEDS, SEE YOUR HEALTH CARE PROFESSIONAL, PREFERABLY A REGISTERED DIETICIAN.

SEDENTARY INDIVIDUALS. Take your current weight and multiply it by the number 9. For example, a 150-pound person should lose weight if he/she consumes no more than 1350 calories per day.

ACTIVE PEOPLE. Take your current weight and multiply it by the number 10. For example a 170-pound person should lose weight if he/she consumes no more than 1700 calories per day.

VERY ACTIVE PEOPLE. Take your current weight and multiply it by the number 12. For example, a 125-pound person should lose weight he/she consumes no more than 1500 calories per day.

IF THE BODY WEIGHT REMAINS STABLE: CALORIES IN = CALORIES OUT

EQUILIBRIUM

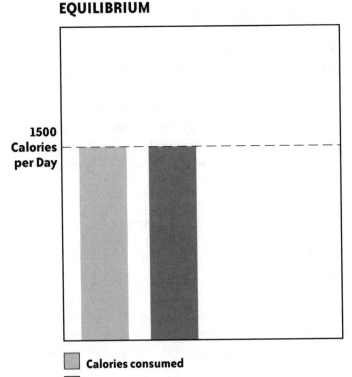

When your body weight is stable, you're expending through your daily activity the same number of calories you consume. This equilibrium (calories in = calories out) is represented by equal height of the two bars in the chart above—this individual is eating and burning off about 1,500 calories every day. Maintaining a stable weight may or may not involve a regular fitness routine. You burn calories with all kinds of activity, though obviously you burn more jogging than you do walking to your car. The less you exercise, the more limited your intake, if you want to maintain your current weight.

THREE WEIGHT-LOSS SCENARIOS

WEIGHT-LOSS SCENARIO #1

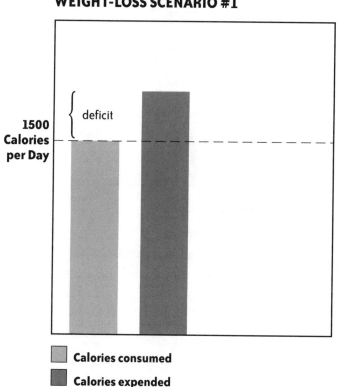

1500 Calories per Day

deficit

Calories consumed

Calories expended

When you devote more time to exercise without increasing the calories you consume, you lose body weight. Calories in dip below calories out, and you've created a deficit. In fact whenever calories burned through exercise exceed the calories you consume, you've got a calorie deficit which leads to weight loss.

WEIGHT-LOSS SCENARIO #2

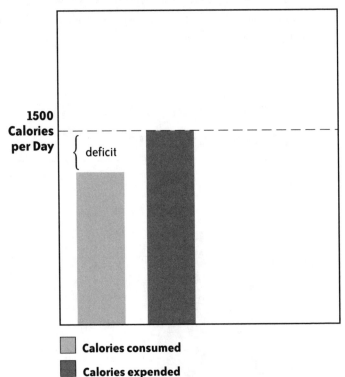

When you decrease food intake while maintaining the same activity level, you lose body weight. Another deficit situation, though weight loss achieved by slashing intake alone is hard to keep off.

WEIGHT-LOSS SCENARIO #3

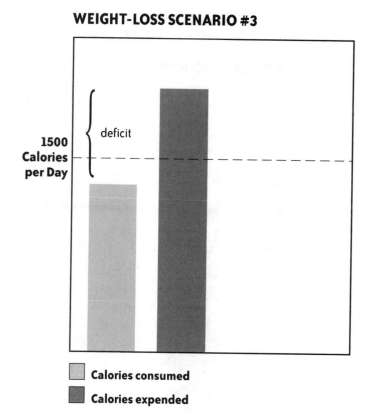

1500 Calories per Day

deficit

■ Calories consumed

■ Calories expended

When you reduce food intake and increase your commitment to exercise, you can lose significant amounts of weight and you're more likely to keep it off.

THREE WEIGHT-GAIN SCENARIOS

WEIGHT-GAIN SCENARIO #1

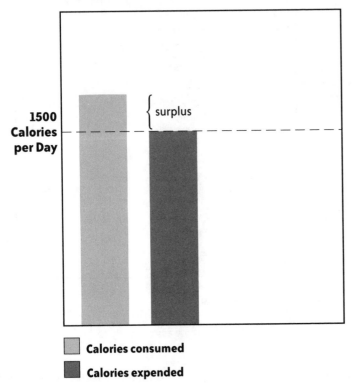

When you increase food intake without expending more calories through exercise, you gain weight, a surplus situation.

WEIGHT-GAIN SCENARIO #2

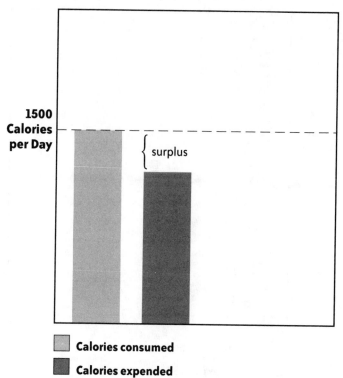

Calories consumed
Calories expended

When you cut back on the time you spend exercising and keep your food intake stable, you gain body weight. Calories in now exceed calories out, and you've created a surplus. Whenever the calories you consume exceed the calories you burn, that surplus will inevitably lead to weight gain.

WEIGHT-GAIN SCENARIO #3

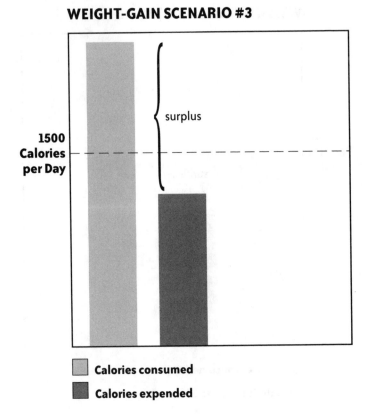

surplus

**1500
Calories
per Day**

■ **Calories consumed**
■ **Calories expended**

If you increase food consumption *and* cut back on exercise, you can gain a lot of weight quickly. Look at that calorie surplus!

LOSING SCALE WEIGHT

To effectively lose weight, you must increase energy expenditure while decreasing calorie consumption. Translated, this means eating less while burning more calories through exercise. In order to lose 1 pound in a week, you must create a 3500-calorie deficit (500 calories less per day). The easiest way to achieve this goal is to adhere to an exercise program that burns roughly 250 calories per day and decrease your caloric intake by 250 calories as well. How much is 250 calories? Well, you can always check food labels, which clearly indicate caloric values, but to give you a general sense of what you're trying to cut out of your daily diet, here's a list of 250-calorie food and beverages:

- One 20-ounce cola or other sugar-sweetened beverage
- 8 candy caramels
- 10 butterscotch hard candies
- 1 Milky Way bar
- ½ large bagel with cream cheese
- 5 Oreo cookies
- ½ cup premium ice cream
- ¾ cup chicken stuffing
- 1¼ cups plain pasta
- 2½ ounces of cheese (2 slices)
- 3 tablespoons peanut butter
- 1 plain biscuit (fast food)
- 25 French fries
- 3 chocolate chunk cookies

You may already recognize that this list doesn't include a significant amount of nutrients. Omitting any of the above items from your diet won't diminish the quality of your dietary intake. At Exude, in New York City, we have found that our clients are most successful with weight loss when they limit these so-called empty calories. In addition to these junk foods, there is a long list of foods considered by many to be healthy which do not contribute significant vitamins or minerals to a diet. Here are some examples:

- White rice
- White pasta
- White bread
- Fructose-sweetened products
- Pretzels

- Baked tortilla chips
- Low-fat baked products (fatfree muffins, cakes, etc.)

There's nothing wrong with these foods except that if they constitute too large a portion of your diet, they can inhibit weight loss. For example, a bagel with no topping may contain 400 to 500 calories. That's more calories than the average person burns during a workout. We at Exude encourage our clients to eat all high-nutrient foods, even if they contain some fat. In the end they will end up consuming fewer calories overall. Our clients often come to us with diets that are *too* low in fat. If you eat too little fat, you will be hungry and feel deprived. And those feelings inevitably lead to the same place—the land of overindulgence.

When you start your eating/exercise program, you should follow these guidelines to the tee. After you have begun to realize your weight loss and fitness goals, you will be able to add a greater variety of food to your diet, but it's a good idea to keep the following in mind:

Foods to Limit

- White breads, cereals with a high sugar content, and white rice (a maximum of 3 servings a week)
- Sugar-sweetened products (frozen yogurt, a maximum of 2 servings a week)
- High-sugar fruits (dried fruits, bananas, fruit juice)
- Desserts—even "low calorie" or "sugarfree"
- Caloric beverages (colas, juices, iced teas, etc.)
- Starchy vegetables (peas, corn, potatoes)
- Saturated fats

Foods to Include

- Lean protein (chicken, fish, low-fat cheese, tofu)
- Low-sugar dairy products (cottage cheese, yogurt, low-fat milk)

- High-fiber breads and cereals, whole grains
- Low-sugar fruits (berries, melon, citrus, plums, peaches, apples)
- Nonstarchy vegetables (lettuce, broccoli, green beans, spinach, mushrooms, onions)
- Sunflower seeds, pumpkin seeds, walnuts
- Low-calorie beverages
- Beans
- Small quantities of monounsaturated and polyunsaturated fats
- Cottage cheese

LET'S TALK SENSE HERE

Eating correctly and exercising properly is paramount in achieving weight loss. Exercising is the *only* way that *anyone* trying to lose and then maintain a lower weight can do it. Exercise is also the only way to naturally and permanently improve your body's proportion of lean mass to fat. Many people who merely diet find that the number on the scale goes down while they still have flabby arms and thighs. This is because the body does not readily burn fat (use fat as a source of fuel). Once your body depletes carbohydrate resources (the body's primary fuel source), it may begin to utilize protein as a source for fuel, leading to the loss of lean mass (muscle). So your weight may go down but you probably won't lose much body fat. By adding proper exercise based on your body type to your lifestyle, your body will begin to burn fat (use fat stores for energy) and "spare" protein. And by exercising properly for your body type you can reduce your fat-to-muscle ratio and sculpt your body into a better-proportioned shape. As muscles are strengthened, you'll burn even more fat and calories, even while you sleep!

Healthy Eating Tips

- The only way to succeed at losing weight and keeping it off is to incorporate permanent healthy eating behavior.

- Decrease the amount of fat in your diet: per gram, fat provides more than twice the calories of carbohydrates and protein.
- Increase fiber (fruits, vegetables, whole grains, dried beans, peas); fiber may actually reduce the amount of calories absorbed by the body.
- Limit bread, rice, potatoes, and pasta—these foods are easy to overeat, contributing to weight gain.
- Limit calorie-containing beverages (soda, juice, alcohol—a piña colada can pack as many as 425 calories).
- Drink 8 to 10 glasses of water every day. Water not only fills you up, helps control your appetite, and increases your energy, it also aids in the metabolism of fat!
- Increase your intake of vegetables: vegetables are low in calories and high in fiber. Look for a variety of bright colors to maximize your nutrient intake.
- *Slow down!* It takes twenty minutes for your brain to receive the message that you're full. You can slow down your meals by taking time to chew every morsel, putting your utensils down between bites, and drinking water throughout the meal.
- Eat bigger at breakfast and lunch and lighter at dinner. By fueling your body with high-fiber low-fat foods during the day, you will avoid overeating at night.
- Make sure each meal contains a low-fat protein source (skinless chicken/turkey, tuna packed in water, soy, low-fat dairy products). Protein aids in satiety and keeps you full longer than carbohydrates.
- Keep a food journal to evaluate your eating patterns. The key is to record what you eat immediately after eating, before you forget. Becoming aware of your food habits is the first step to changing them so you can succeed at weight loss.

Healthy Snacking

Going for long periods of time without eating usually results in extreme hunger, the number one stimulus for overeating. Snacking between meals can help keep you energized throughout the day and keep hunger away, making it easier to stick to your weight-loss regimen. Keep in mind that snacking in between meals can result in weight gain if you eat too many calories overall.

Healthy Choices for Low-Fat Snacks Include:

- 2 graham crackers + 1 teaspoon jam
- 1 ounce of reduced-fat cheese with 10 whole-wheat crackers
- 1 slice of muenster cheese melted over tomato on whole-wheat bread
- Non-fat yogurt with 2 tablespoons low-fat granola
- Protein bar or shake (check food label: 200 calories and no more than 7 grams of fat!)
- 1 ounce low-fat shredded cheese melted over 1 medium-baked potato
- ¼ cup dry-roasted mixed nuts (almonds, pumpkin seeds, walnuts)
- ½ cup trail mix (dried fruit, pretzels, nuts, cereal)
- 1 cup fruit salad with ½ cup low-fat cottage cheese
- ½ whole-wheat English muffin + 1 slice low-fat mozzarella + 1 tablespoon marinara sauce
- 3 egg whites + salsa rolled into a whole wheat tortilla
- 1 medium orange diced into 1 serving of oatmeal

SUMMARY

Your diet and nutrition needs are far more complicated than your exercise needs. You might not relish exercise, but no one's literally allergic to it. There are, however, millions of people who cannot and/or should not eat certain foods. Sometimes it's difficult to detect food allergies. You can eat a particular food for years without recognizing that it's bad for you. Because we eat more often than we exercise, there is simply a lot more room for error. For many, eating is an emotional crutch. Stress and other factors in our lives affect our eating patterns and cravings and the amount of food that we consume. All that is to say that figuring out what and how much to eat is far from simple. That is why I have not outlined a specific eating plan, menus or recipes here. It would be as long if not longer than this book. If you find yourself not able to lose weight with the information I've provided, then please make an appointment with a registered dietician and seek out his or her expert advice.

What I will say is that whether it's social or emotional, we tend to be extreme in our eating patterns. Either we eat like gluttons or eat like birds. Moderation is not in our vocabulary. Sadly, sound fitness programs and sensible, nutritious eating habits aren't instilled in us as children. I cannot emphasize enough the importance of paying attention to your child's activity level and eating habits. Statistically, if they are obese or vastly overweight as children, then as adults they will become only worse. So, if you do have a child or children who are gravitating toward inactivity or obesity, seek professional help immediately—don't wait! We all need to learn to say no to our children (especially when we're saying no to junk food or a second dessert) and realize it's okay. For those who do need additional help in this area or regarding other issues concerning your children, I highly suggest you consult the work of noted expert of parent-child communication Dr. Norma Ross (www.youcansayno.com). Her insight, perspective and advice will enlighten the way you look at parenting just as I hope I have impacted you when it comes to motivational fitness.

Finally, I want you to be patient and honest with yourself. If you look in the mirror and like what you see and feel, great, fine. But if you don't like what you see, stop complaining and start making the changes necessary to become your best. I've never met anyone who exercises for his or her body type and eats sensibly who doesn't exude beauty, health, confidence and energy. So get off your duff and do whatever it takes to get it done. I promise that you will live a more complete and productive and a happier and longer life!

Note that sections of this chapter were created with the help of Hillary Baron, M.S., RD.

## PART II

THE BODY-TYPE WORKOUTS

Before you choose one of the body-type workouts to follow, there are a few things you must
know and do in order to capitalize on your efforts. First, each of the body types has three
core workouts and an off-day routine—the beginner core workout (for those who are sedentary), the active core workout and the advanced
workout. I suggest strongly that unless you
are currently working out at least 4 days per
week and performing some kind of a full-body
fitness routine, start either at the beginner
or active level. Most of the exercises will be totally new to both your body and your mind.
When you feel you can increase the intensity, switch over to the active or advanced workout. If you cannot complete the recommended
number of repetitions for a particular exercise,
keep track of the number you *can* do. With

time, you will work up to the recommended number and then surpass it.

No matter what your body type, the better shape you're in, the more intensely you should be exercising. So if you're in good shape, start pushing yourself a few minutes into your warm-up. Don't just warm up at a leisurely pace. Challenge yourself because you will reap aerobic benefits and burn more calories! If you are having trouble with your form, body alignment or coordination, I highly recommend you exercise in front of a mirror, which will help you see what mistakes you're making and correct them quickly.

All of the workouts are full-body exercise regimes that address and hit all 5 components of fitness and follow American College of Sports Medicine guidelines by including the 4 phases with each workout as well. If you want to speed up the process and need to lose more weight and mass, follow the off-day routines between workouts.

If you experience any aches, pains or minor strains during your workout, stop immediately. That's the *end* of your workout for that day. Ice the area and use an ace bandage to support it. Don't resume until you are feeling better. If the pain persists after a few days, see your doctor. *Do not* heat injured muscles for the first 72 hours. Stick to the ice! If you are having difficulty performing *any* of the exercises, including jumping rope, you may contact us (see page 270) for help.

Below are some rules and guidelines to follow that will aid you in escaping your shape.

Rules of the Game

- Be consistent and work out 3 to 5 days per week.
- Take your measurements prior to your first workout, then once every 30 days thereafter.
- Complete all four essential phases of a workout—warm-up, stretch, workload, and cooldown—every time you work out!

- Don't do any other workout on the days in between, especially if it is contraindicated for your body type. If you want to exercise more often than when I prescribe, follow the off-day routines.
- Do not substitute *any* of the exercises within your workout unless there's a medical or orthopedic reason to do so. It's essential that you perform exercises that are right for your body type in order to see results.
- Perform all of the exercises in the *exact* order prescribed, even if you can't complete the recommended number of repetitions. No skipping!
- Even if you don't like a particular exercise, do it anyway. With time, your body will start to change and you'll come to like all of them—because you'll get better and better at them.
- Don't ask your "trainer" or anyone else for his or her opinion on any of the exercises. If they knew anything, your body would have changed already and you wouldn't have bought this book!
- If you travel, stay at hotels that offer access to fitness equipment, at least a stationary bike or treadmill. The rest you can take with you.
- As you become more fit, increase the intensity of your workouts. This will ensure that your body will continue to improve.
- Purchase a good pair of cross-training sneakers and use them only for your body-type workouts.
- Never work out in bare feet unless you take a jog on the beach.
- When you're jumping rope, avoid double jumping (jumping twice for each turn of the rope). Keep your feet close to the ground.
- Do not work out within two hours of eating a full meal. Make sure you do not exercise unless you have eaten at least a small meal one or two hours prior to beginning your workout.
- Drink small amounts of water (about ½ cup, 4 ounces) every 10 or 20 minutes during your workout. Do not drink huge quantities of water before or during your workout. It is best to drink water often but in small amounts.
- Don't hold your breath during any stretches or exercises. Breathe through your mouth and not through your nose.

## CHAPTER 7

The Hourglass Workout

Welcome, Hourglasses! Most Hourglasses who come to me for help are trying to lose weight, mass and inches from both their upper and lower bodies. Specifically, they want to slim, tone and streamline their hips, thighs and upper arms. Each core workout should be performed 3 days per week and should take you about 60 minutes to complete. If you want to speed up the toning process or have excess weight to shed, I recommend you perform your off-day routine at least 2 days per week in addition to your core workouts. For example, you might choose Mondays, Wednesdays and Fridays as your core workout days and throw in an off-day routine on Tuesdays and Saturdays. Don't schedule two core workouts on consecutive days. Your body needs time to rest and recover. You can, however, perform back-to-back off-day routines.

TOOLS NEEDED
Women

- Stationary bike or treadmill*
- 4-pound aerobic bar (for both upper and lower body)
- Exercise mat
- Jump rope

Men

- Stationary bike or treadmill*
- 4-pound aerobic bar (for lower body)
- 10- to 15-pound weighted bar (for upper body)
- Exercise mat
- Jump rope

* Please note: If you do not HAVE ACCESS TO A STATIONARY BIKE OR A TREADMILL, YOU CAN WALK OR MARCH IN PLACE FOR THE AEROBIC PORTIONS OF YOUR WORKOUT (OR SEE BODY TYPE AND AEROBIC FITNESS EQUIPMENT CHART, PAGE 50).

AEROBIC AND ANAEROBIC INTERVALS

As an Hourglass, you want to perform as much aerobic exercise as you can, especially if you're trying to lose weight and mass. The *key* is to keep the resistance/tension as low as possible for both your upper and lower bodies. Challenge yourself by increasing the RPMs or MPHs on the stationary bike or treadmill as you bike, walk or run. Remember, the bigger you are, the lower the resistance or tension setting should be. As you start to lose weight and mass, you can increase your resistance/tension ever so slightly. If your body is medically and orthopedically sound, I have found the jump rope to be the most effective tool for losing weight and trimming the upper arms, back and lower body. If you're not able to jump rope, the next best thing is a recumbent stationary bike. Hourglass women who need to tone their upper and lower bodies should use nothing heavier than a 4-pound aerobic bar. It's light enough to tone you without bulking any region of your body.

Men should start out with the 10-pound curl bar for all upper-body exercises. As you trim down, you can switch to a 12- or 15-pound bar. If you're happy with your scale weight but need to lose inches and to tone, cut back on your aerobic exercise and focus on calisthenics and bar exercises for both the upper and lower bodies. Keep in mind that as an Hourglass you need to keep the resistance/tension low or moderate and the repetitions high so that you do not bulk. With a heavier bar or high resistance, you may firm up but not lose the inches you hope to. If this is the case, return to the lighter bar and lighter resistance for all of your exercises and add more repetitions. That should do the trick.

INCREASING YOUR INTENSITY

As an Hourglass, it's important to increase the intensity of your upper- and lower-body exercises in order to escape your shape. Say when you start out on the stationary bike, you're riding at 50 to 70 RPMs and your heart rate is 150 beats per minute (BPM). If you stick to a consistent workout schedule, in just two weeks you'll have markedly improved your fitness level. You can measure how much by checking your heart rate, which will have dropped to around 130 BPM. Now it's time to intensify your workout, in your case by increasing your *speed*, not *resistance*. In doing so, you'll burn more calories and see steady progression toward your weight-loss goals. Whatever you do, avoid increasing the resistance/tension for either your upper- or lower-body exercises until you've slimmed down; otherwise you will stop losing inches or, worse yet, start to bulk! Don't worry, increasing your speed alone will ramp up your workout intensity effectively. You can also cut back on breaks between exercises and sets and add more repetitions. If jumping rope is a part of your workout, try turning the jump rope faster and incorporating footwork into your jump rope intervals. You'll burn more calories and improve your fitness level, not to mention impress your friends and family. . . .

I can't say this too many times—you need to keep increasing the intensity of your workouts until you are totally satisfied with your body and fitness level. Remember, you won't reach your goals unless you get mentally tough and ramp up your workouts so that they continue to challenge you. Extending your warmup and aerobic intervals are ways to effectively increase your intensity, but if you're like many of my clients, finding that extra time can be more challenging than the physical task at hand. Instead, you can speed up your aerobic activity and/or add repetitions to your anaerobic routine. Of the two—extending the length of your workout versus increasing speed and adding repetitions—the latter is more effective and efficient. You'll burn more calories and boost your fitness level at the same time.

You can also increase the intensity of your workout by reversing the order of the exercises in your workload. This is recommended only for those of you who have completely mastered each and every exercise in the advanced-core workout. After you warm up and stretch, do your workload in reverse order, ending, of course, with the cooldown.

Please note: Hourglass workouts are patent pending.

BEGINNER CORE WORKOUT

The beginner core workout should be done 3 times per week, with each session lasting approximately 40 to 50 minutes.

1. **WARM-UP:** 10 to 20 minutes
   - **Bike** at 50 to 70 RPMs, with low tension **OR**
   - **Walk** (with or without treadmill) at 2.7 to 3.2 MPH with no incline

2. **STRETCH:** 2 to 4 minutes. Perform each stretch for 30 to 60 seconds.
   - **Arm Circles:** Stand up straight, knees slightly flexed, feet shoulder-width apart. With arms outstretched, slowly circle your arms forward for 5 revolutions. Make as large a circle as you can. Then reverse and circle your arms backward for 5 revolutions.

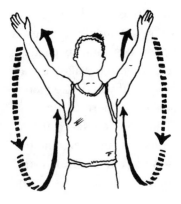

- **Triceps:** With arms straight overhead, bend your right arm so that your right elbow is behind your head. Place your left palm on your right elbow and gently press that elbow toward the wall behind you until you feel the stretch in your shoulder and triceps. Switch arms and repeat.

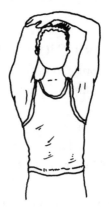

- **Upper Back and Chest Stretch:** Bend forward at the waist, with knees slightly bent. Grasp your hands behind your back, then lift your arms up and hold until you feel a good stretch in your chest and in the front of your shoulders and upper arms.

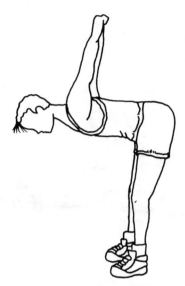

- **Spine Twist:** Sit with both legs extended straight in front of you. Cross your right leg over your left, placing your right foot flat on the floor to the left of your left knee. Turn your upper body clockwise (to the right) and place your right hand palm down on the floor behind you. With your left elbow or hand pressing against the outside of your right knee, turn your torso as far to the right (clockwise) as you can as you look over your right shoulder. Reverse arms and legs, twisting your torso to the left (counterclockwise).

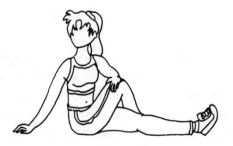

- **Hamstrings:** Sit with your legs extended straight in front of you. Bend forward from the hips and reach for your toes. If you can, grab your toes and hold.

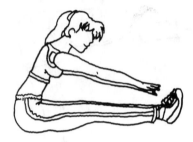

- **Legs-Apart Hamstrings:** Sit with your legs extended and spread as far apart as you can. Bend forward at the hips, moving your hands toward your ankles. Grab your ankles (or the top of your shoes, if you can), gently pull your upper body forward and hold.

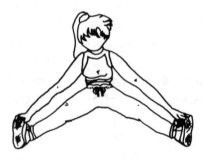

- **Groin:** In a seated position, bring the soles of your shoes together and hold them in place by grabbing your ankles. Gently pull your heels toward your groin. Let your knees relax toward the mat, then press your elbows down on your knees to increase the stretch. Hold when you feel the stretch in your inner thigh and groin.

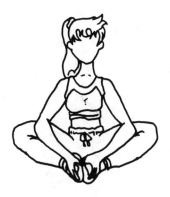

- **Quadriceps:** Lie down on your right side. Bend your left leg back and grab your left ankle with your left hand. Gently pull your leg back toward your buttocks. Hold when you feel a comfortable stretch in the front of your thigh. Release and roll over onto your left side and repeat.

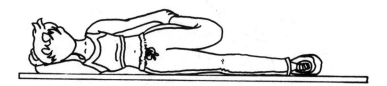

- **Calves:** Stand with your right leg forward and bent at the knee, your left leg fully extended behind you. Place both hands palms flat up against a wall and lean forward. Think about pressing your left heel into the floor. Hold. Then switch legs and repeat.

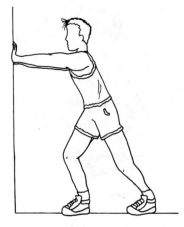

- **Calves (Alternative):** Get down on all fours. Straighten your legs, keeping your palms flat on the floor in front of you. Press your right heel down toward the floor while your left heel is off the floor, left toe touching the floor. After stretching the right calf, switch positions so that you are now pressing the heel of your left foot toward the floor while your right heel is off the floor.

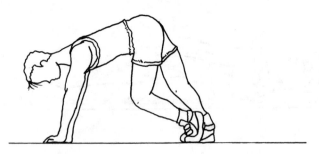

3. **AEROBIC INTERVAL:** 3 minutes
   - **Bike** at 60+ RPMs **OR**
   - **Walk** at 3.2 MPH

4A. STANDING KNEE TO OPPOSITE CHEST (with a 4-pound aerobic bar): 15 per leg

Rest the bar on your neck across your shoulders, with feet shoulder-width apart. Transfer all weight to your right leg. Raise your left knee up toward your right chest to at least waist level. Lower your left foot to the starting position. Your weight stays centered on your right leg throughout the movement. Repeat 14 times, then switch legs.

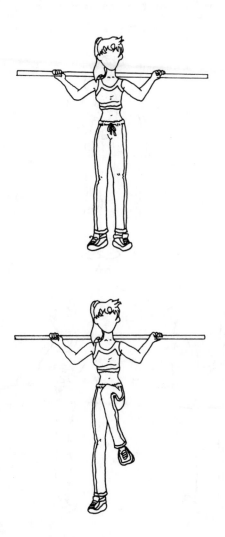

4B. L-KICKS: 15 per leg

Hold the aerobic bar upright with your right hand and place your left hand on your waist. Starting with your left leg, point your toe and gently raise your left leg straight in front of you as high as possible. Use the bar to help you balance, but don't lean on it. Return to the starting position, lightly touching the ground. Now raise the left leg to the side as high as possible. Again, no leaning on the bar. Repeat 14 times, then switch legs and repeat.

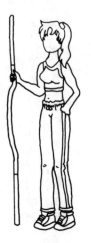

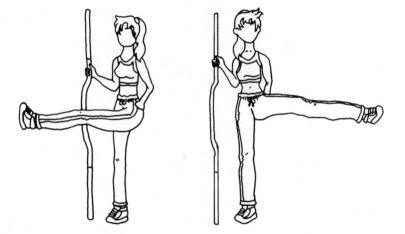

5. AEROBIC INTERVAL: 3 minutes
- **Bike** at 60+ RPMs *OR*
- **Walk** at 3.2 MPH

6. UPPER-BODY ROUTINE (with a 4-pound aerobic bar for women or a weighted bar for men): 15 reps for each exercise with no rest in between exercises
- **Push-outs:** Keep your back straight, knees slightly flexed and feet shoulder-width apart. Grip aerobic bar, palms facing down, just wider than shoulder-width apart. Raise bar up just above your chest line with elbows up and wrists firm. Extend arms straight out, holding bar above chest level as you exhale. Keeping arms straight, lower bar to the front of your thighs. Inhale while you raise your arms for the next rep, exhale as you push out. Keep entire body aligned and still.

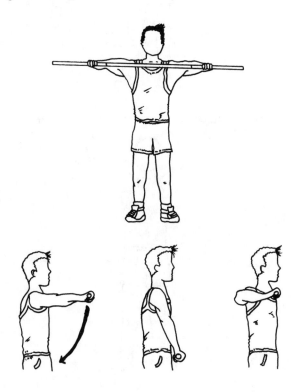

- **Behind-the-Neck Press:** Keep back straight, knees flexed and feet shoulder-width apart. Grip aerobic bar with palms facing outward just wider than shoulder-width apart and rest it lightly on your shoulders behind your neck. Extend your arms straight up while exhaling. Now bend your arms, lowering the bar to the start position as you inhale.

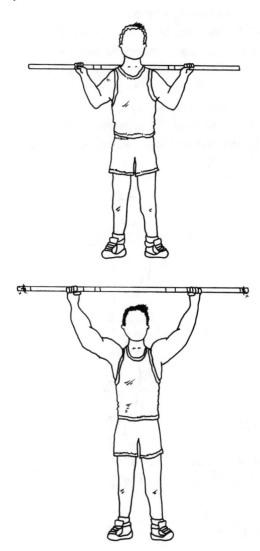

- **Front Press:** Keep back straight, knees flexed and feet shoulder-width apart. Grip aerobic bar with palms facing outward just wider than shoulder-width apart and rest bar across top of chest. Extend your arms, raising the bar straight up while you exhale. Bend your arms and slowly return bar to the start position as you inhale.

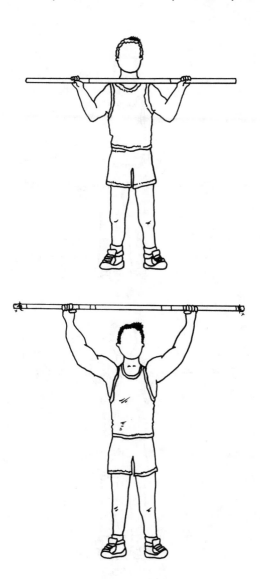

- **Upright Rows:** Keep back straight, knees flexed and feet shoulder-width apart. Grip aerobic bar, palms facing down, hands 6 to 12 inches apart. Hold bar with arms fully extended against the front of your thighs. Slowly raise bar toward your chin, keeping elbows above bar level as you exhale. Return to the start position as you inhale.

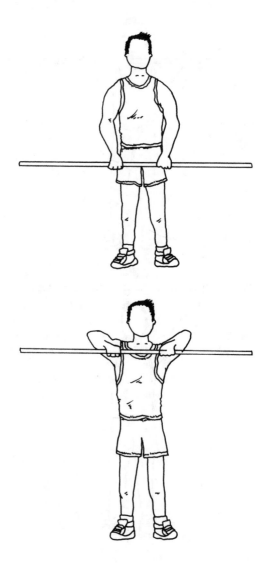

- **Bicep Curl:** Keep back straight, knees flexed and feet shoulder-width apart. Grip aerobic bar, palms facing up, hands shoulder-width apart. Hold bar with arms fully extended against the front of your thighs. Keeping wrists firm and elbows at your side, curl the bar up to your chest as you exhale. Slowly return bar to the start position as you inhale.

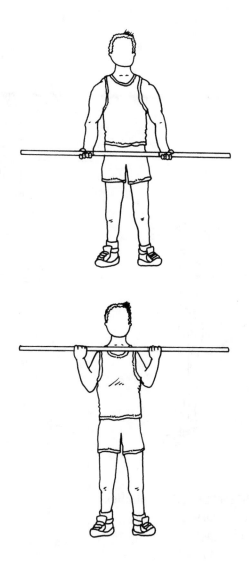

- **Tricep Kickbacks:** Keep back straight, knees flexed and feet shoulder-width apart. Grip aerobic bar behind your back. Start with the bar resting lightly against the buttocks, palms facing outward. Keeping elbows and wrists firm, raise the bar up and back as you exhale. Keeping arms straight, lower bar to the start position as you inhale.

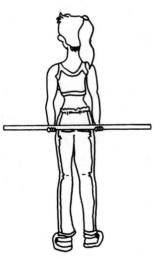

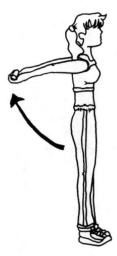

7. **AEROBIC INTERVAL:** 3 minutes
   - **Bike** at 60+ RPMs *OR*
   - **Walk** at 3.2 MPH

8. **ABDOMINALS, HIPS AND THIGHS:** 10 to 20 reps each with 30 seconds rest in between exercises.

- **Sit-ups:** Lie on your back with knees bent, feet flat on the floor, fingertips at your temples. Slowly raise your head and shoulders off the ground until your elbows touch your knees as you exhale. Lower to the starting position and inhale. For an easier sit-up, perform with arms fully extended, as shown below.

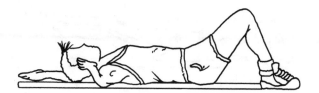

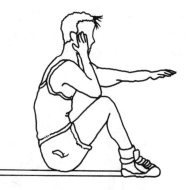

- **Leg-outs:** Lie on your back, with hands under your buttocks, palms down, and bring both knees in toward your chest. Slowly straighten legs out with toes pointed. Inhale while bringing knees toward chest, exhale as you straighten your legs. Beginners can raise their legs higher, but as your abdominals grow stronger, try lowering your legs closer to the mat.

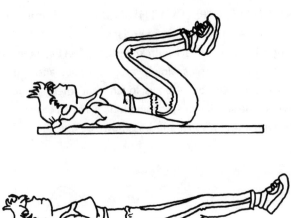

- **Vertical Scissors:** Lie on your back, hands at your sides, palms down. Raise your legs to a 90-degree angle. Pressing your back into the floor and with toes pointed, slowly open your legs as wide as you can. Bring legs back together, keeping toes pointed as you exhale.

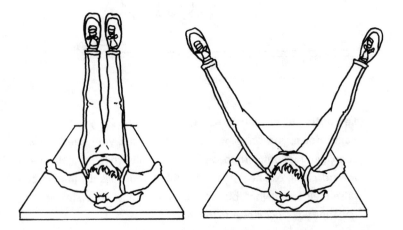

- **Alternate Leg Raises:** Lie on your back with your hands under your buttocks, palms down. Raise your right leg to a 90-degree angle, your left remaining on the floor. Pressing the small of your back into the floor, lower your right leg as you simultaneously lift your left leg. Repeat this continuous scissoring motion.

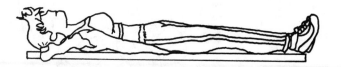

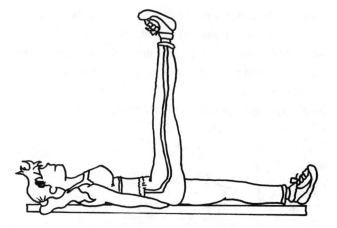

- **Elbows to Knees:** Lie on your back. Raise knees and feet toward your chest. Clasp your hands together at the base of your neck, then curl your upper body, bringing your elbows to your knees. Slowly lower your upper body to the mat. The lower half of your body remains motionless. Exhale as you bring elbows to knees.

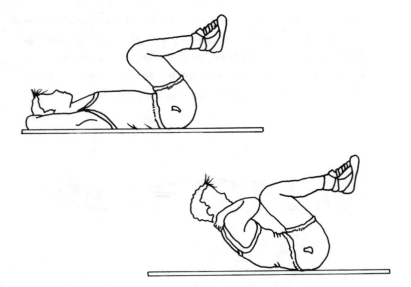

- **Knees to Elbows:** Lie on the floor with hands clasped at the base of your neck. Raise your head and shoulders off the floor. Your upper body remains in this position. Now raise your knees and feet in a tucked position toward your elbows, keeping your lower back pressed to the floor. Lower your toes to the ground, then exhale as you raise knees to elbows to begin the next rep.

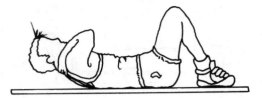

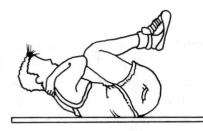

9. **REPEAT UPPER-BODY ROUTINE** (with a 4-pound aerobic bar for women or a weighted bar for men): 10 to 15 reps for all exercises with no rest in between
   - Push-outs
   - Behind-the-Neck Press
   - Front Press
   - Upright Rows
   - Bicep Curls
   - Tricep Kickbacks

10. **AEROBIC INTERVAL:** 3 minutes
   - **Bike** at 60+ RPMs *OR*
   - **Walk** at 3.2 MPH

11. **COOLDOWN:** 2 to 3 minutes
   - **Bike** leisurely *OR*
   - **Walk**

BEGINNER OFF-DAY ROUTINE

This off-day routine is to be performed in conjunction with your body-type workout. It is designed for those who are seeking to lose weight and/or add additional workouts to their exercise regime. I advise you to perform 2 or 3 off-day routines per week until you've slimmed down to your ideal weight, then ease up and go to 1 or 2 days per week thereafter. This routine should take approximately 30 to 40 minutes to complete.

1. **WARM-UP:** 20 to 30 minutes
   - **Bike** at 60+ RPMs *OR*
   - **Walk** at 3.0 MPH

2. **STRETCH:** 2 to 4 minutes. Perform each stretch for 30 to 60 seconds.
   - Arm Circles
   - Triceps

- Upper Back and Chest Stretch
- Spine Twist
- Hamstrings
- Legs-Apart Hamstrings
- Groin
- Quadriceps
- Calves

3. **JUMPING JACKS:** Do 25, bike or walk for 1 minute to catch your breath, then repeat.

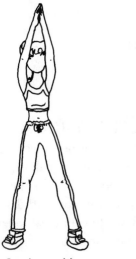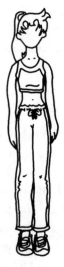

Starting position

4. **COOLDOWN:** 2 to 3 minutes
   - **Bike** leisurely **OR**
   - **Walk**

ACTIVE CORE WORKOUT

If you're in pretty good shape to begin with, you may want to start with this more advanced workout, or you can ramp up to it when you're ready to increase the intensity of your workout. This workout should be done 3 times per week, with each session lasting approximately 60 minutes. All exercises are illustrated in the beginner core workout.

1. **WARM-UP:** 10 to 20 minutes
   - **Bike** at 70 to 90 RPMs with low tension *OR*
   - **Walk** (with or without a treadmill) at 3.0 to 3.5 MPH

2. **STRETCH:** 2 to 4 minutes. Perform each stretch for 30 to 60 seconds.
   - Arm Circles
   - Triceps
   - Upper Back and Chest Stretch
   - Spine Twist
   - Hamstrings
   - Legs-Apart Hamstrings
   - Groin
   - Quadriceps
   - Calves

3. **AEROBIC INTERVAL:** 5 minutes
   - **Bike** at 80+ RPMs *OR*
   - **Walk** at 3.5 MPH *OR*
   - **Jump rope** for 100 jumps, then bike or walk for 3 minutes

4. **STANDING KNEE TO OPPOSITE CHEST** (with a 4-pound aerobic bar): 25 per leg

5. **L-KICKS** (with 4-pound aerobic bar): 25 per leg

6. **AEROBIC INTERVAL:** 5 minutes
   - **Bike** at 80+ RPMs *OR*
   - **Walk** at 3.5 MPH *OR*
   - **Jump rope** for 100 jumps, then bike or walk for 3 minutes

7. **UPPER-BODY ROUTINE** (with a 4-pound aerobic bar for women or a weighted bar for men): 25 reps of each, no breaks in between exercises
   - Push-outs
   - Behind-the-Neck Press
   - Front Press
   - Upright Row
   - Curls
   - Tricep Kickbacks

8. **AEROBIC INTERVAL:** 5 minutes
   - **Bike** at 80+ RPMs *OR*
   - **Walk** at 3.5 MPH *OR*
   - **Jump rope** for 100 jumps, then bike or walk for 3 minutes

9. **ABDOMINALS, HIPS AND THIGHS:** 30 reps each with 10 seconds rest in between exercises
   - Sit-ups
   - Leg-outs
   - Vertical Scissors
   - Alternate Leg Raises
   - Elbows to Knees
   - Knees to Elbows

10. **UPPER-BODY ROUTINE** (with a 4-pound aerobic bar for women or a weighted bar for men): 15 reps each
    - Push-outs
    - Behind-the-Neck Press
    - Front Press
    - Upright Row
    - Curls
    - Tricep Kickbacks

11. AEROBIC INTERVAL: 5 minute
- **Bike** at 80+ RPMs *OR*
- **Walk** at 3.5 MPH *OR*
- **Jump rope** for 100 jumps, then bike or walk for 3 minutes

12. COOLDOWN: 2 to 3 minutes
- **Bike** leisurely *OR*
- **Walk**

ACTIVE OFF-DAY ROUTINE

This off-day routine is to be performed in conjunction with your body-type workout. It is designed for those who are seeking to lose weight and/or add additional workouts to their exercise regime. I advise you to perform 2 or 3 off-day routines per week until you've slimmed down to your ideal weight, then ease up and go to 1 or 2 days per week thereafter. This routine should take approximately 45 minutes to complete. All exercises are illustrated in the beginner core workout.

1. WARM-UP: 30 minutes
- **Bike** at 80+ RPMs *OR*
- **Walk** at 3.5+ MPH

2. STRETCH: 2 to 4 minutes. Perform each stretch for 30 to 60 seconds.
- Arm Circles
- Triceps
- Upper Back and Chest Stretch
- Spine Twist
- Hamstrings
- Legs-Apart Hamstrings
- Groin
- Quadriceps
- Calves

3. **AEROBIC INTERVAL:**
   - **Do 50 jumping jacks,** then bike or walk for 1 minute to catch your breath **OR**
   - **Jump rope** for 100 jumps, than bike or walk for 1 minute to catch your breath

4. **STANDING KNEE TO OPPOSITE CHEST** (with a 4-pound aerobic bar): 25 per leg

5. **L-KICKS** (with a 4-pound aerobic bar): 25 per leg

6. **AEROBIC INTERVAL:**
   - **Do 50 jumping jacks,** then bike or walk for 1 minute to catch your breath **OR**
   - **Jump rope** for 100 jumps, then bike or walk for 1 minute to catch your breath.

7. **COOLDOWN:** 2 to 3 minutes
   - **Bike** leisurely **OR**
   - **Walk**

ADVANCED CORE WORKOUT

This workout should be done 3 times per week, with each session lasting approximately 60 minutes. All exercises are illustrated in the beginner core workout.

1. **WARM-UP:** 10 to 20 minutes
   - **Bike** at 90 to 110+ RPMs with low tension **OR**
   - **Walk** (with or without treadmill) at 3.5 to 4.2 MPH

2. **STRETCH:** 2 to 4 minutes. Perform each stretch for 30 to 60 seconds.
   - Arm Circles
   - Triceps
   - Upper Back and Chest Stretch

- Spine Twist
- Hamstrings
- Legs-Apart Hamstrings
- Groin
- Quadriceps
- Calves

3. **AEROBIC INTERVAL:** 3 minutes
   - **Bike** at 90+ RPMs *OR*
   - **Walk** at 4.2 MPH *OR*
   - **Jump rope** for 200 jumpss

4. **STANDING KNEE TO OPPOSITE CHEST** (with a 4-pound aerobic bar): 35 per leg

5. **L-KICKS:** 35 per leg

6. **AEROBIC INTERVAL:** 3 minutes
   - **Bike** at 90+ RPMs *OR*
   - **Walk** at 4.2 MPH *OR*
   - **Jump rope** for 200 jumps

7. **UPPER-BODY ROUTINE** (with a 4-pound aerobic bar for women or a weighted bar for men): 40 reps each with no rest in between
   - Push-outs
   - Behind-the-Neck Press
   - Front Press
   - Upright Rows
   - Curls
   - Tricep Kickback

8. **AEROBIC INTERVAL:** 3 minutes
   - **Bike** at 90+ RPMs *OR*
   - **Walk** at 4.2 MPH *OR*
   - **Jump rope** for 200 jumps

9. **ABDOMINALS, HIPS AND THIGHS:** 50 reps each with 10 seconds rest in between exercises
   - Sit-ups
   - Leg-outs
   - Vertical Scissors
   - Alternate Leg Raises
   - Elbows to Knees
   - Knees to Elbows

10. **UPPER-BODY ROUTINE** (with a 4-pound aerobic bar for women or a weighted bar for men): 25 reps for all exercises with no rest in between exercises
    - Push-outs
    - Behind-the-Neck Press
    - Front Press
    - Upright Rows
    - Curls
    - Tricep Kickbacks

11. **AEROBIC INTERVAL:** 3 minutes
    - **Bike** at 90+ RPMs **OR**
    - **Walk** at 4.2 MPH **OR**
    - **Jump rope** for 200 jumps

12. **COOLDOWN:** 2 to 3 minutes
    - **Bike** leisurely **OR**
    - **Walk**

ADVANCED OFF-DAY ROUTINE

This off-day routine is to be performed in conjunction with your body-type workout. It is designed for those who are seeking to lose weight and/or add additional workouts to their exercise regime. I advise you to perform 2 or 3 off-day routines per week until you've slimmed down to your ideal weight, then ease up and go to 1 or 2 days per week thereafter. This routine should take approximately 45 minutes to complete.

1. **WARM-UP:** 20 minutes
   - **Bike** at 90+ RPMs *OR*
   - **Walk** at 4.0+ MPH

2. **STRETCH:** 2 to 4 minutes. Perform each stretch for 30 to 60 seconds.
   - Arm Circles
   - Triceps
   - Upper Back and Chest Stretch
   - Spine Twist
   - Hamstrings
   - Legs-Apart Hamstrings
   - Groin
   - Quadriceps
   - Calves

3. **AEROBIC INTERVAL:**
   - **Do 75 to 100 jumping jacks *OR***
   - **Jump rope** for 2 minutes, then
   - **Bike or walk** for 1 minute to catch your breath

4. **STANDING KNEE TO OPPOSITE CHEST** (with a 4-pound aerobic bar): 50 per leg

5. **L-KICKS** (with a 4-pound aerobic bar): 35 per leg

6. **AEROBIC INTERVAL:**
   - **Do 75 to 100 jumping jacks *OR***
   - **Jump rope** for 2 minutes *OR*
   - **Bike or walk** for 1 minute to catch your breath

7. **ABDOMINALS, HIPS AND THIGHS:** 50 reps for each with no rest in between exercises
   - Sit-ups
   - Leg-outs
   - Vertical Scissors
   - Alternate Leg Raises

- Elbows to Knees
- Knees to Elbows

8. **AEROBIC INTERVAL:**
   - **Do 75 to 100 jumping jacks OR**
   - **Jump rope** for 2 minutes **OR**
   - **Bike or walk** for 1 minute to catch your breath

9. **COOLDOWN:** 2 to 3 minutes
   - **Bike** leisurely **OR**
   - **Walk**

MOVING FORWARD

As you progress and get in better shape, you want to work up to a full 3 minutes of jumping rope for each 3-minute aerobic interval. When you can jump rope for four 3-minute intervals within your workout, try jumping rope for 5 to 10 minutes for your first and last intervals, and eliminate the second and third intervals altogether. It should take you 30 to 60 days to work up to 10 minutes of jumping rope. By incorporating different footwork into your jump intervals, you'll work different muscle groups and increase your intensity. If you cannot jump rope because of a medical or orthopedic concern, then bike vigorously instead! Your goal is to work up to 50 to 100 repetitions for each exercise and to jump rope continuously for 30 minutes without taking a break.

If your goal is to lose weight and inches and you find after 45 days of working out you are losing inches but not scale weight, then you need to adjust your diet or the frequency of workouts or both (see Chapter 6). The *key* to your success is to be consistent, to work hard and to focus on performing all of the exercises even if you cannot at first do the number of recommended repetitions. With time you will be able to do even the advanced workout without a hitch.

## CHAPTER 8

The Spoon Workout

If you're anything like the Spoons who come to Exude for help, your goal is to transform your body from a ladle to a little teaspoon! As Spoons, you're more than likely targeting the hips, thighs and saddlebag region of your body for slimming. You'll also want to strengthen your upper body. Each core workout should be performed 3 days per week and should take you about 60 minutes to complete. If you want to speed up the toning process or have excess weight to shed, I recommend you perform your off-day routine at least 2 days per week in addition to your core workouts. For example, you might choose Mondays, Wednesdays and Fridays as your core workout days and throw in an off-day routine on Tuesdays and Saturdays. Don't schedule two core workouts on consecutive days. Your body needs time to rest and recover. You can, however, perform back-to-back off-day routines.

TOOLS NEEDED
Women

- Stationary bike or treadmill*
- 4-pound aerobic bar
- 10-pound curl bar
- Exercise mat
- Jump rope

Men

- Stationary bike or treadmill*
- 4-pound aerobic bar
- 10- to 15-pound weighted bar
- Exercise mat
- Jump rope

* PLEASE NOTE: IF YOU DO NOT HAVE ACCESS TO A STATIONARY BIKE OR A TREAD-MILL, YOU CAN WALK OR MARCH IN PLACE FOR THE AEROBIC PORTIONS OF YOUR WORKOUT (OR SEE BODY TYPE AND AEROBIC FITNESS EQUIPMENT CHART, PAGE 50).

AEROBIC AND ANAEROBIC INTERVALS

I cannot emphasize enough the importance of reviewing the recommended exercises and the exercises that as a Spoon you should stay away from. For your lower body, *make sure* that the resistance/tension settings on all aerobic equipment are low; if you feel you need to challenge yourself, knock yourself out by jacking up the speed or RPMs. No squats or lunges! For your upper body, unless you're 10 or more pounds overweight, use moderate to high resistance/tension. You don't bulk as easily up top and you want to add strength and a little mass there, anyway. If you are overweight, I suggest you start out using the 4-pound aerobic bar for your upper-body exercises. After you have lost weight, you can move up to the 10-pound curl bar. Men should use the 10- to 15-pound straight bar for their upper-body exercises regardless of current weight.

The more weight and mass you need to lose, the more aerobic exercise you need to perform. As you approach your ideal weight, you can do a little less aerobic exercise and increase the amount of anaerobic exercises, such as your upper-body routine and calisthenics. The most effective way to take mass off your lower body is to jump rope. For those who cannot jump rope because of medical or orthopedic conditions, use a recumbent stationary bike. Performing your off-day routine will speed up your weight loss—and you'll lose inches faster, too. Remember, your goal is not to necessarily bulk up your upper body to match the size of your lower body, but rather to lose weight and mass down below and to strengthen your upper body. Additional muscle mass above will help your body look more proportionate. As a Spoon, it's important to remember that even after you lose weight or mass below, you need to stay away from high-resistance/tension exercises for the rest of your exercise life—that goes for *all* lower-body aerobic and anaerobic exercises.

INCREASING YOUR INTENSITY

Whether you're walking, riding the stationary bike, or jumping rope—all Spoon-preferred aerobic exercises—it's important to keep increasing your intensity to ensure that your lower body continues to change. Don't make the mistake of increasing intensity by increasing the resistance/tension. That will only bulk you up down below. The speed at which you bike (RPMs), walk (MPH) or jump rope (revolutions/jumps per minute) is what you need to focus on. You'll also want to increase the number of reps for your mat work and hip/thigh exercises. For your upper body, you can add more weight to your routine (so long as you are not overweight) or add other sets here and there within your core workout. Work extra hard on those push-ups! Most female Spoons don't like doing push-ups because—at least at first—they are so difficult for them. Be patient and work through it. Within 30 days or so, they'll be much easier and you'll see significant improvements. For those who can jump rope, try varying your footwork, which also raises the intensity of your workout, burns more calories and improves your fitness level. You want to build up to 150 revolutions per minute and work up to 30 minutes of continuous jumping without taking a single break. Taking fewer, shorter breaks in between exercises and sets will increase intensity as well. If you cannot jump rope because of a medical or orthopedic concern, aim for biking at high speeds (100+ RPMs). As a Spoon, your best friends are the bike, the rope and the hip/thigh exercises using the 4-pound aerobic bar.

As you become better conditioned, you need to be more aggressive with your warm-up as well. You can either extend the duration of your warm-up, jog or bike faster, or both. I recommend my clients go for speed. It's hard to make extra time, and besides, it's much more beneficial fitness-wise to increase the intensity. As you master the beginner and active workouts and move toward the advanced workouts, you can also reverse the order of the exercise in your workout, ending, of course, with a cooldown.

Please note: Spoon workouts are patent pending.

BEGINNER CORE WORKOUT

The beginner core workout should be done 3 times per week, with each session lasting approximately 40 to 50 minutes.

1. **WARM-UP:** 10 to 20 minutes
   - **Bike** at 50+ RPMs with low tension **OR**
   - **Walk** (with or without treadmill) with no incline at 3.0+ MPH

2. **STRETCH:** 2 to 4 minutes. Perform each stretch for 30 to 60 seconds.
   - **Arm Circles:** Stand up straight, knees slightly flexed, feet shoulder-width apart. With arms outstretched, slowly circle your arms forward for 5 revolutions. Make as large a circle as you can. Then reverse and circle your arms backward for 5 revolutions.

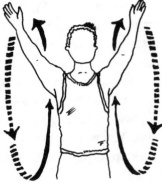

- **Triceps:** With arms straight overhead, bend your right arm so that your right elbow is behind your head. Place your left palm on your right elbow and gently press that elbow toward the wall behind you until you feel the stretch in your shoulder and triceps. Switch arms and repeat.

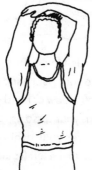

- **Upper Back and Chest Stretch:** Bend forward at the waist, with knees slightly bent. Grasp your hands behind your back, then lift your arms up and hold until you feel a good stretch in your chest and in the front of your shoulders and upper arms.

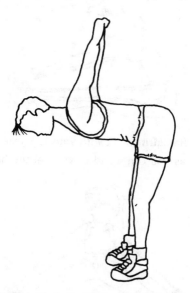

- **Spine Twist:** Sit with both legs extended straight in front of you. Cross your right leg over your left, placing your right foot flat on the

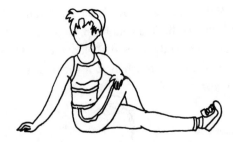

floor to the left of your left knee. Turn your upper body clockwise (to the right) and place your right hand palm down on the floor behind you. With your left elbow or hand pressing against the outside of your right knee, turn your torso as far to the right (clockwise) as you can as you look over your right shoulder. Reverse arms and legs, twisting your torso to the left (counterclockwise).

- **Hamstrings:** Sit with your legs extended straight in front of you. Bend forward from the hips and reach for your toes. If you can, grab your toes and hold.

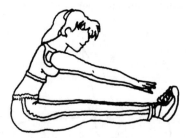

- **Legs-Apart Hamstrings:** Sit with your legs extended and spread as far apart as you can. Bend forward at the hips, moving your

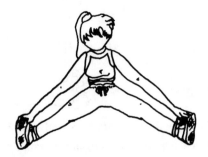

hands toward your ankles. Grab your ankles (or the top of your shoes, if you can); gently pull your upper body forward and hold.

- **Groin:** In a seated position, bring the soles of your shoes together and hold them in place by grabbing your ankles. Gently pull your heels toward your groin. Let your knees relax toward the mat, then press your elbows down on your knees to increase the stretch. Hold when you feel the stretch in your inner thigh and groin.

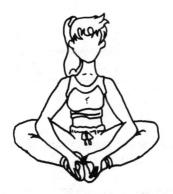

- **Quadriceps:** Lie down on your right side. Bend your left leg back and grab your left ankle with your left hand. Gently pull your leg back toward your buttocks. Hold when you feel a comfortable stretch in the front of your thigh. Release and roll over onto your left side and repeat.

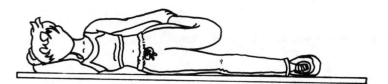

- **Calves:** Stand with your right leg forward and bent at the knee, your left leg fully extended behind you. Place both hands palms

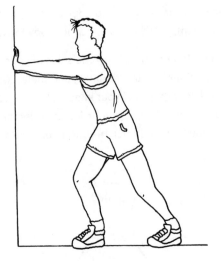

flat up against a wall and lean forward. Think about pressing your left heel into the floor. Hold. Then switch legs and repeat.

- **Calves (Alternative):** Get down on all fours. Straighten your legs, keeping your palms flat on the floor in front of you. Press your right heel down toward the floor while your left heel is off the floor, left toe touching the floor. After stretching the right calf, switch foot positions so that you are now pressing the heel of your left foot toward the floor while your right heel is off the floor.

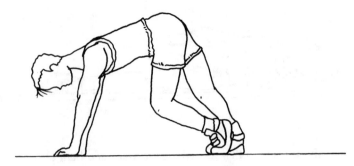

3. **STANDING KNEE TO OPPOSITE CHEST** (with a 4-pound aerobic bar): 20 per leg

Rest the aerobic bar on your neck across your shoulders, with feet shoulder-width apart. Transfer all weight to your right leg. Raise your left knee up toward your right chest to at least waist level. Lower your left foot to the starting position. Your weight stays centered on your right leg throughout the movement. Repeat 14 times, then switch legs.

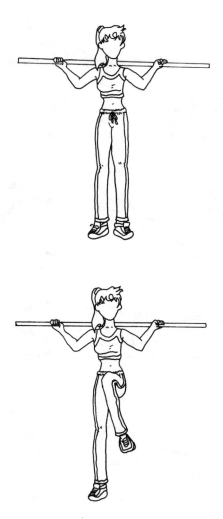

4. PUSH-UPS: 5 to 10 on either knees or toes

Start on hands and knees with your ankles crossed (or on your hands and toes). Hands should be slightly wider than shoulder-width apart, fingers pointing forward, and tummy in. Inhale as you lower your chest as close to the floor as possible. Exhale as you push up to the starting position. Do not lock your elbows. Gradually build to 25.

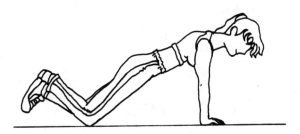

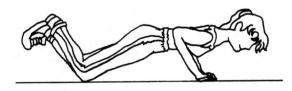

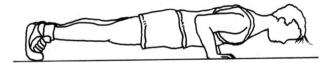

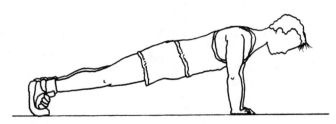

5. AEROBIC INTERVAL: 3 minutes
- **Bike** at 70 RPMs *OR*
- **Walk** at 3.0+ MPH

6. UPPER-BODY ROUTINE (with a 10-pound curl bar for women or a 10- to 15-pound weighted bar for men): 20 reps for each exercise with 10-second rests in between exercises.
- **Push-outs:** Keep your back straight, knees slightly flexed and feet shoulder-width apart. Grip bar, palms facing down, just wider than shoulder-width apart. Raise bar up just above your chest line with elbows up and wrists firm. Extend arms straight out, holding bar above chest level as you exhale. Keeping arms straight, lower bar to the front of your thighs. Inhale while you raise your arms for the next rep, exhale as you push out. Keep entire body aligned and still.

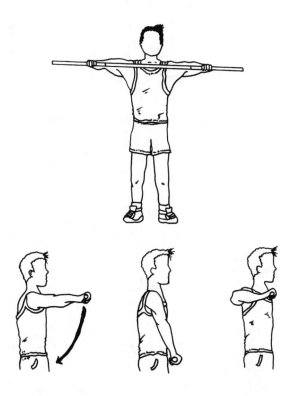

- **Behind-the-Neck Press:** Keep back straight, knees flexed and feet shoulder-width apart. Grip bar with palms facing outward just wider than shoulder-width apart and rest it lightly on your shoulders behind your neck. Extend your arms straight up while exhaling. Now bend your arms, lowering the bar to the start position as you inhale.

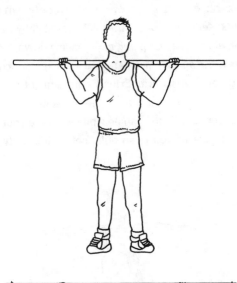

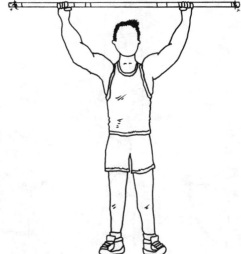

- **Front Press:** Keep back straight, knees flexed and feet shoulder-width apart. Grip bar with palms facing outward just wider than shoulder-width apart and rest bar across top of chest. Extend your arms, raising the bar straight up while you exhale. Bend your arms and slowly return bar to the start position as you inhale.

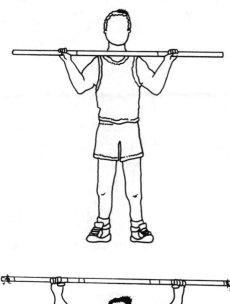

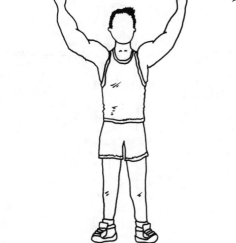

- **Upright Rows:** Keep back straight, knees flexed and feet shoulder-width apart. Grip bar, palms facing down, hands 6 to 12 inches apart. Hold bar with arms fully extended against the front of your thighs. Slowly raise bar toward your chin, keeping elbows above bar level as you exhale. Return to the start position as you inhale.

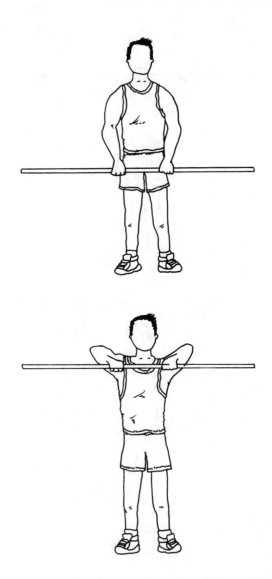

- **Bicep Curl:** Keep back straight, knees flexed and feet shoulder-width apart. Grip bar, palms facing up, hands shoulder-width apart. Hold bar with arms fully extended against the front of your thighs. Keeping wrists firm and elbows at your side, curl the bar up to your chest as you exhale. Slowly return bar to the start position as you inhale.

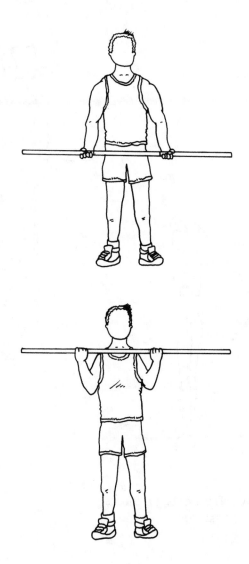

- **Tricep Kickbacks:** Keep back straight, knees flexed and feet shoulder-width apart. Grip bar behind your back. Start with the bar resting lightly against the buttocks, palms facing outward. Keeping elbows and wrists firm, raise the bar up and back as you exhale. Keeping arms straight, lower bar to start position as you inhale.

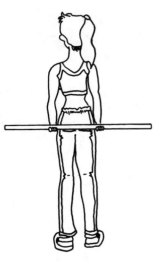

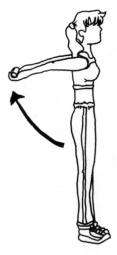

7. **AEROBIC INTERVAL:** 3 minutes
   - **Bike** at 70 RPMs **OR**
   - **Walk** at 3.0+ MPH

8. ABDOMINALS, HIPS AND THIGHS: 25 reps each with 30 seconds rest in between exercises

- **Sit-ups:** Lie on your back with knees bent, feet flat on the floor, fingertips at your temples. Slowly raise your head and shoulders off the ground until your elbows touch your knees as you exhale. Lower to the starting position and inhale. For an easier sit-up, perform with arms fully extended, as shown below.

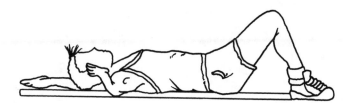

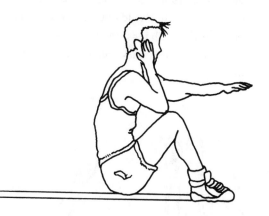

- **Leg-outs:** Lie on your back, with hands under your buttocks, palms down, and bring both knees in toward your chest. Slowly straighten legs out with toes pointed. Inhale while bringing knees toward chest; exhale as you straighten your legs. Beginners can raise their legs higher, but as your abdominals grow stronger, try lowering your legs closer to the mat.

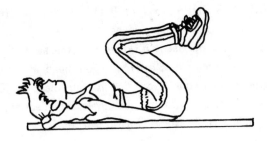

- **Vertical Scissors:** Lie on your back, hands at your sides, palms down. Raise your legs to a 90-degree angle. Pressing your back into the floor and with toes pointed, slowly open your legs as wide as you can. Bring legs back together, keeping toes pointed as you exhale.

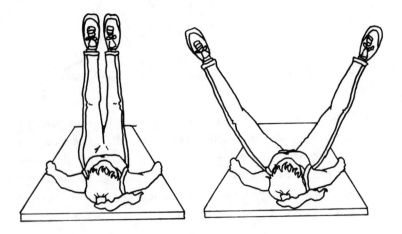

- **Alternate Leg Raises:** Lie on your back with your hands under your buttocks, palms down. Raise your right leg to a 90-degree angle, your left remaining on the floor. Pressing the small of your back into the floor, lower your right leg as you simultaneously lift your left leg. Repeat this continuous scissoring motion.

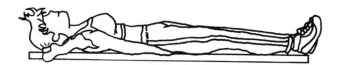

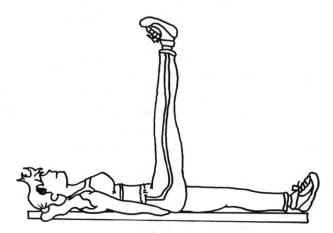

- **Repeat Leg-outs**

- **Repeat Alternate Leg Raises**

- **Elbows to Knees:** Lie on your back. Raise knees and feet toward your chest. Clasp your hands together at the base of your neck, then curl your upper body, bringing your elbows to your knees. Slowly lower your upper body to the mat. The lower half of your body remains motionless. Exhale as you bring elbows to knees.

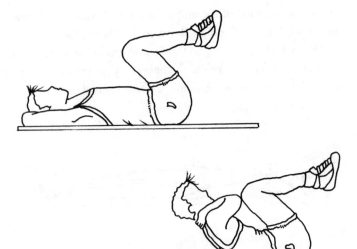

- **Knees to Elbows:** Lie on the floor with hands clasped at the base of your neck. Raise your head and shoulders off the floor. Your upper body remains in this position. Now raise your knees and feet in a tucked position toward your elbows, keeping your lower back pressed to the floor. Lower your toes to the ground, then exhale as you raise knees to elbows to begin the next rep.

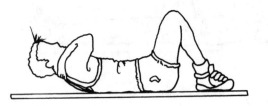

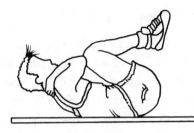

9. STANDING KNEE TO OPPOSITE CHEST (with a 4-pound aerobic bar): 20 per leg

Rest the aerobic bar on your neck across your shoulders, with feet shoulder-width apart. Transfer all weight to your right leg. Raise your left knee up toward your right chest to at least waist level. Lower your left foot to the starting position. Your weight stays centered on your right leg throughout the movement. Perform 20 reps, then switch legs.

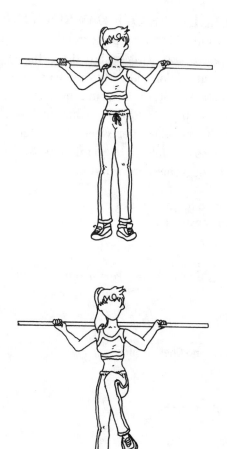

10. AEROBIC INTERVAL: 3 minutes
- **Bike** at 70 RPMs *OR*
- **Walk** at 3.0+ MPH

11. COOLDOWN: 2 to 3 minutes
- **Bike** leisurely *OR*
- **Walk**

BEGINNER OFF-DAY ROUTINE

This off-day routine is to be performed in conjunction with your body-type workout. It is designed for those who are seeking to lose weight and/or add additional workouts to their exercise regime. I advise you to perform 2 or 3 off-day routines per week until you've slimmed down to your ideal weight, then ease up and go to 1 or 2 days per week thereafter. This workout should take approximately 30 to 40 minutes. All exercises are illustrated in the beginner core workout.

1. WARM-UP: 20 to 30 minutes
- **Bike** at 60+ RPMs *OR*
- **Walk** at 3.0 MPH

2. STRETCH: 2 to 4 minutes. Perform each stretch for 30 to 60 seconds.
- Arm Circles
- Triceps
- Upper Back and Chest Stretch
- Spine Twist
- Hamstrings
- Legs-Apart Hamstrings
- Groin
- Quadriceps
- Calves

3. STANDING KNEE TO OPPOSITE CHEST (with a 4-pound aerobic bar): 20 reps

4. L-KICKS: 15 per leg

Hold the aerobic bar upright with your right hand and place your left hand on your waist. Starting with your left leg, point your toe and gently raise your left leg straight in front of you as high as possible. Use the bar to help you balance, but don't lean on it. Return to the starting position, lightly touching the ground. Now raise the left leg to the side as high as possible. Again, no leaning on the bar. Repeat 14 times, then switch legs and repeat.

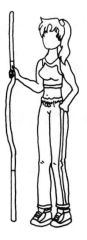

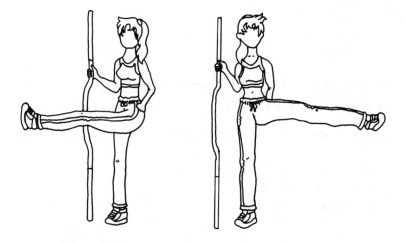

5. **COOLDOWN:** 2 to 3 minutes
   - **Bike** leisurely *OR*
   - **Walk**

ACTIVE CORE WORKOUT

If you're in pretty good shape to begin with, you may want to start with this more advanced workout, or you can ramp up to it when you're ready to increase the intensity of your workout. This workout should be done 3 times per week, with each session lasting approximately 45 minutes. All exercises are illustrated in the beginner core workout.

1. **WARM-UP:** 10 to 20 minutes
   - **Bike** at 70+ RMPs with low tension *OR*
   - **Walk** (with or without treadmill) with no incline at 3.5+ MPH

2. **STRETCH:** 2 to 4 minutes. Perform each stretch for 30 to 60 seconds.
   - Arm Circles
   - Triceps
   - Upper Back and Chest Stretch
   - Spine Twist
   - Hamstrings
   - Legs-Apart Hamstrings
   - Groin
   - Quadriceps
   - Calves

3. **STANDING KNEE TO OPPOSITE CHEST** (with a 4-pound aerobic bar): 30 for each leg

4. **PUSH-UPS:** 10 to 20 on either knees or toes

5. **AEROBIC INTERVAL:** 5 minutes
   - **Bike** at 80+ RPMs *OR*
   - **Walk** at 3.5 MPH

6. UPPER-BODY ROUTINE: 35 reps each
- Push-outs
- Behind-the-Neck Press
- Front Press
- Upright Rows
- Curls
- Tricep Kickbacks

7. AEROBIC INTERVAL: 3 minutes
- **Bike** at 70 RPMs *OR*
- **Walk** at 3.0+ MPH

8. ABDOMINALS, HIPS AND THIGHS: 40 reps each with 10 seconds rest in between exercises
- Sit-ups
- Leg-outs
- Vertical Scissors
- Alternate Leg Raises
- Elbows to Knees
- Knees to Elbows

9. STANDING KNEE TO OPPOSITE CHEST (with a 4-pound aerobic bar): 30 per leg

10. AEROBIC INTERVAL: 3 minutes
- **Bike** at 80+ RPMs *OR*
- **Walk** at 3.5 MPH

11. COOLDOWN: 2 to 3 minutes
- **Bike** leisurely *OR*
- **Walk**

Please note: You may substitute jumping rope for biking or walking during aerobic intervals.

ACTIVE OFF-DAY ROUTINE

This off-day routine is to be performed in conjunction with your body-type workout. It is designed for those who are seeking to lose weight and/or add additional workouts to their exercise regime. I advise you to perform 2 or 3 off-day routines per week until you've slimmed down to your ideal weight, then ease up and go to 1 or 2 days per week thereafter. This routine should take approximately 30 to 40 minutes to complete. All exercises are illustrated in the beginner core workout.

1. **WARM-UP:** 30 minutes
   - **Bike** at 80 RPMs **OR**
   - **Walk** at 3.5+ MPH with no incline

2. **STRETCH:** 2 to 4 minutes. Perform each stretch for 30 to 60 seconds.
   - Arm Circles
   - Triceps
   - Upper Back and Chest Stretch
   - Spine Twist
   - Hamstrings
   - Legs-Apart Hamstrings
   - Groin
   - Quadriceps
   - Calves

3. **JUMP ROPE:** 3 to 5 minutes, going back and forth to bike or walk when you need to catch your breath

4. **STANDING KNEE TO OPPOSITE CHEST** (with a 4-pound aerobic bar): 30 reps per leg

5. **JUMP ROPE:** 3 to 5 minutes, going back and forth to bike or walk when you need to catch your breath

6. **COOLDOWN:** 2 to 3 minutes
   - **Bike** leisurely **OR**
   - **Walk**

ADVANCED CORE WORKOUT

This workout should be done 3 times per week, with each session lasting approximately 60 minutes. All exercises are illustrated in the beginner core workout.

1. **WARM-UP:** 10 to 20 minutes
   - **Bike** at 90+ RPMs with low tension **OR**
   - **Walk** (with or without treadmill) with no incline at 4.0 + MPH

2. **STRETCH:** 2 to 4 minutes. Perform each stretch for 30 to 60 seconds.
   - Arm Circles
   - Triceps
   - Upper Back and Chest Stretch
   - Spine Twist
   - Hamstrings
   - Legs-Apart Hamstrings
   - Groin
   - Quadriceps
   - Calves

3. **STANDING KNEE TO OPPOSITE CHEST** (with a 4-pound aerobic bar): 40 per leg

4. **PUSH-UPS:** 20 to 30 on either knees or toes

5. **AEROBIC INTERVAL:** 3 minutes
   - **Jump rope** (200 jumps), then
   - **Bike** at 90+ RPMs or walk at 4.0 MPH for the remainder of the 3 minutes

6. **UPPER-BODY ROUTINE:** 50 reps each exercise with no rest in between exercises
   - Push-outs
   - Behind-the-Neck Press

- Front Press
- Upright Rows
- Curls
- Tricep Kickbacks

7. AEROBIC INTERVAL: 3 minutes
- **Jump rope** (200 jumps), then
- **Bike** at 90+ RPMs or walk at 4.0 MPH for the remainder of the 3 minutes

8. ABDOMINALS, HIPS AND THIGHS: 50 reps each with no rest in between exercises
- Sit-ups
- Leg-outs
- Vertical Scissors
- Alternate Leg Raises
- Elbows to Knees
- Knees to Elbows

9. STANDING KNEE TO OPPOSITE CHEST (with a 4-pound aerobic bar): 40 per leg

10. AEROBIC INTERVAL: 3 minutes
- **Jump rope** (200 jumps) *OR*
- **Bike** at 90+ RPMs or walk at 4.0 MPH for the remainder of the 3 minutes

11. COOLDOWN: 2 to 3 minutes
- **Bike** leisurely *OR*
- **Walk**

ADVANCED OFF-DAY ROUTINE

This off-day routine is to be performed in conjunction with your body-type workout. It is designed for those who are seeking to lose weight and/or add additional workouts to their exercise regime. I advise you to perform 2 or 3 off-day routines per week until you've slimmed down to your ideal weight, then ease up and go to 1 or 2 days per week thereafter. This routine should take approximately 45 minutes to complete. All exercises are illustrated in the beginner core workout.

1. WARM-UP: 20 minutes
- **Bike** at 100+ RPMs *OR*
- **Walk** at 4.0+ MPH with no incline

2. STRETCH: 2 to 4 minutes. Perform each stretch for 30 to 60 seconds.
- Arm Circles
- Triceps
- Upper Back and Chest Stretch
- Spine Twist
- Hamstrings
- Legs-Apart Hamstrings
- Groin
- Quadriceps
- Calves

3. JUMP ROPE: 5 to 10 minutes, going back and forth to bike or walk when you need to catch your breath

4. STANDING KNEE TO OPPOSITE CHEST (with a 4-pound aerobic bar): 40 per leg

5. JUMP ROPE: 5 to 10 minutes, going back and forth to bike or walk when you need to catch your breath

6. COOLDOWN: 2 to 3 minutes

MOVING FORWARD

As you improve your cardiovascular health and stamina, you should work up to a full 3 minutes of jumping rope for *each* 3-

minute aerobic interval. When you can jump three 3-minute intervals within your workout, try jumping rope for 5 to 10 minutes for your first and last intervals, and eliminate the second
interval of jumping altogether. It should take you 30 to 60 days
to build up to 10 minutes of jumping rope, sooner if you perform your off-day routine more than twice a week. If you cannot jump rope due to medical or orthopedic constraints, bike
vigorously instead for all of the aerobic intervals. Spoons, it's essential that you remember to increase intensity selectively—
jack up the speed but not the resistance/tension for *all*
lower-body exercises. You'll also want to increase the weight
you use and the number of sets/repetitions you perform for all
of your upper-body exercises. Your goal is to work up to 100
repetitions for all anaerobic exercises and to bike at 110 + RPMs
or walk at 4.5 MPH.

If you want to lose both weight and inches and find that after
45 days or so that you are losing inches but not scale weight,
you may need to adjust your diet or the frequency of your workouts (see Chapter 6). Focus on being consistent. When you eat
or drink a little bit more than you should, counter that with
extra aerobic intervals or an additional off-day workout that
week. Until you can perform all of the recommended exercises
and repetitions for the beginner and active workouts, don't skip
ahead to the very active workouts. Don't worry, with consistent
and dedicated exercise, you will master even the most advanced
workout.

CHAPTER 9

The Ruler Workout

Welcome, all Rulers. Your goal is to reduce your midsection and taper your waist. You need to be especially vigilant about weight gain because most of it goes right to your stomach, creating the illusion that you're much fatter than you actually are. If you're less than 10 pounds overweight, you're lucky—you need only to exercise 3 times per week. On the other hand, if you are carrying more than 10 unwanted pounds, at least one off-day routine will be a part of your weekly workout schedule until that weight is gone.

Find time to do your core workouts 3 times a week. Each session will take approximately 60 minutes. Your workout schedule might look like this: core workouts Mondays, Wednesdays and Fridays plus an off-day workout on Saturday if you are overweight or would like to speed things up. You can do up to three off-day workouts per week, but be sure to allow for a day of rest between core workouts. Your body needs time to recover. You can, however, perform back-to-back off-day workouts on consecutive days.

TOOLS NEEDED
Women

- Stationary bike, treadmill, elliptical or stepper*
- 4-pound aerobic bar
- 10-pound curl bar
- Exercise mat
- Jump rope

Men

- Stationary bike, treadmill, elliptical or stepper*
- 4-pound aerobic bar
- 15-pound straight bar
- Exercise mat
- Jump rope

* PLEASE NOTE: IF YOU DO NOT HAVE ACCESS TO A STATIONARY BIKE OR A TREADMILL, YOU CAN WALK OR MARCH IN PLACE FOR THE AEROBIC PORTIONS OF YOUR WORKOUT (OR SEE BODY TYPE AND AEROBIC FITNESS EQUIPMENT CHART, PAGE 50).

AEROBIC AND ANAEROBIC INTERVALS

Most Rulers divide their workouts evenly between aerobic- and anaerobic-type exercises. Unless you're overweight, you should spend 50 percent of your workout on a bike, stepper or treadmill and the other 50 percent on your abdominals, arms and legs. If you need to lose a little mass, then either incorporate once or twice a week an off-day routine into your schedule or extend the aerobic intervals within your core workout. During your anaerobic work, you want to focus on strengthening your abdominals, back and upper body. You may also want to spend a little extra time stretching your hamstrings, which will help protect your back. As a Ruler, you can perform virtually any exercise without fear of bulking unless you're overweight. And after you shed some pounds, you can perform *all* of your exercises with moderate to high resistance/tension. Rulers make good runners, so if you enjoy it, go for it! You don't need to avoid inclines the way Hourglasses and Spoons do. Additional abdominal work, such as side benders, will help taper your midsection and protect your back—often a weak spot for your body type.

INCREASING INTENSITY

Since most Rulers have to work out only 3 or 4 days per week, the proper intensity level is paramount to your success. As a Ruler, you can choose to increase the intensity of your workouts in any number of ways. For starters you can increase the resistance/tension on all of your aerobic exercises. That is, raise the incline on the treadmill while you walk or jog, or increase the tension on a stationary bike or elliptical trainer. You can also ramp up your speed at the same time as you increase resistance/tension, which will burn even more calories. Remember, as a Ruler you don't have to worry about bulking up unless you're overweight.

Once you can perform 50 reps of your upper-body exercises with either a 10- or 15-pound weight bar, you have a choice. You can either go up in weight in 2- to 5-pound increments (which will build muscle mass) or add more repetitions (if you're happy with the size of your arms and upper body). Performing your dead lifts with additional weight on your core workout days will help strengthen your hamstrings and give your rear end a nice rounding out.

Taking fewer breaks between exercises will also help raise your intensity. Really focus on proper form in your abdominal work and push yourself during your warmup whether you're biking, running or using some other piece of aerobic equipment. You'll improve your fitness level, burn more calories, and maximize the aerobic benefits of your routine without extending your workout.

Please note: Ruler workouts are patent pending.

BEGINNER CORE WORKOUT

The beginner core workout should be done 3 times per week, with each session lasting approximately 40 to 50 minutes.

1. **WARM-UP:** 10 to 20 minutes
   - **Bike** at 50+ RPMs with moderate tension **OR**
   - **Walk** (with or without treadmill) on a slight incline at 2.7 MPH **OR**
   - **Use an elliptical or stepper** with moderate resistance

2. **STRETCH:** 2 to 4 minutes. Perform each stretch for 30 to 60 seconds.
   - **Arm Circles:** Stand up straight, knees slightly flexed, feet shoulder-width apart. With arms outstretched, slowly circle your arms forward for 5 revolutions. Make as large a circle as you can. Then reverse and circle your arms backward for 5 revolutions.

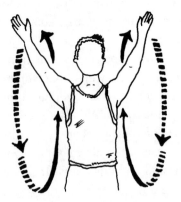

   - **Triceps:** With arms straight overhead, bend your right arm so that your right elbow is behind your head. Place your left palm on your right elbow and gently press that elbow toward the wall behind you until you feel the stretch in your shoulder and triceps. Switch arms and repeat.

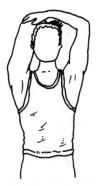

- **Upper Back and Chest Stretch:** Bend forward at the waist, with knees slightly bent. Grasp your hands behind your back, then lift your arms up and hold until you feel a good stretch in your chest and in the front of your shoulders and upper arms.

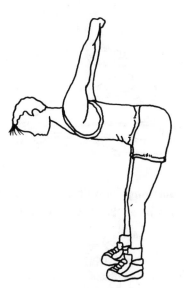

- **Spine Twist:** Sit with both legs extended straight in front of you. Cross your right leg over your left, placing your right foot flat on the floor to the left of your left knee. Turn your upper body clockwise (to the right) and place your right hand palm down on the floor behind you. With your left elbow or hand pressing against the out-

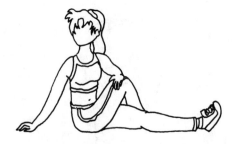

side of your right knee, turn your torso as far to the right (clock-wise) as you can as you look over your right shoulder. Reverse arms and legs, twisting your torso to the left (counterclockwise).

- **Hamstrings:** Sit with your legs extended straight in front of you. Bend forward from the hips and reach for your toes. If you can, grab your toes and hold.

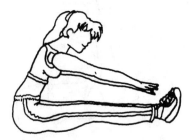

- **Legs-Apart Hamstrings:** Sit with your legs extended and spread as far apart as you can. Bend forward at the hips, moving your

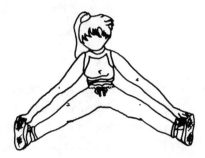

hands toward your ankles. Grab your ankles (or the top of your shoes, if you can), gently pull your upper body forward and hold.

- **Groin:** In a seated position, bring the soles of your shoes together and hold them in place by grabbing your ankles. Gently pull your heels toward your groin. Let your knees relax toward the mat, then press your elbows down on your knees to increase the stretch. Hold when you feel the stretch in your inner thigh and groin.

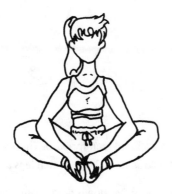

- **Quadriceps:** Lie down on your right side. Bend your left leg back and grab your left ankle with your left hand. Gently pull your leg back toward your buttocks. Hold when you feel a comfortable stretch in the front of your thigh. Release and roll over onto your left side and repeat.

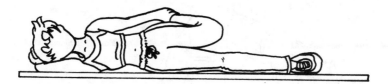

- **Calves:** Stand with your right leg forward and bent at the knee, your left leg fully extended behind you. Place both hands palms

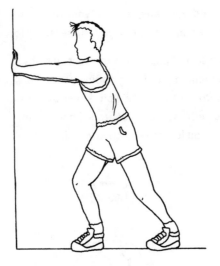

flat up against a wall and lean forward. Think about pressing your left heel into the floor. Hold. Then switch legs and repeat.

- **Calves (Alternative):** Get down on all fours. Straighten your legs, keeping your palms flat on the floor in front of you. Press your right heel down toward the floor while your left heel is off the floor, left toe touching the floor. After stretching the right calf, switch foot positions so that you are now pressing the heel of your left foot toward the floor while your right heel is off the floor.

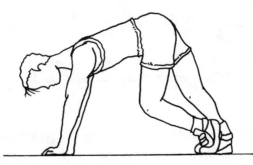

3. ABDOMINALS, HIPS AND THIGHS: 20 of each

- **Sit-ups:** Lie on your back with knees bent, feet flat on the floor, fingertips at your temples. Slowly raise your head and shoulders off the ground until your elbows touch your knees as you exhale. Lower to the starting position and inhale. For an easier sit-up, perform with arms fully extended, as shown below.

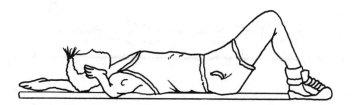

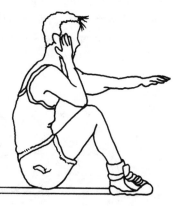

- **Leg-outs:** Lie on your back, with hands under your buttocks, palms down, and bring both knees in toward your chest. Slowly straighten legs out with toes pointed. Inhale while bringing knees toward chest, exhale as you straighten your legs. Beginners can raise their legs higher, but as your abdominals grow stronger, try lowering your legs closer to the mat.

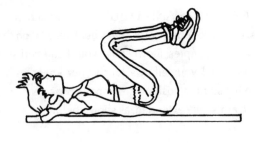

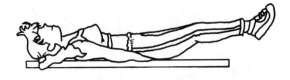

- **Elbows to Knees:** Lie on your back. Raise knees and feet toward your chest. Clasp your hands together at the base of your neck, then curl your upper body, bringing your elbows to your knees. Slowly lower your upper body to the mat. The lower half of your body remains motionless. Exhale as you bring elbows to knees.

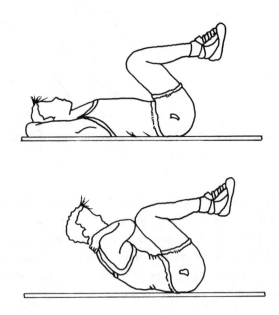

- **Knees to Elbows:** Lie on the floor with hands clasped at the base of your neck. Raise your head and shoulders off the floor. Your upper body remains in this position. Now raise your knees and feet in a tucked position toward your elbows, keeping your lower back pressed to the floor. Lower your toes to the ground, then exhale as you raise knees to elbows to begin the next rep.

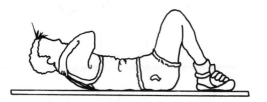

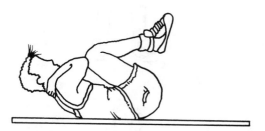

- **Sit-ups (yes, again!)**

4. AEROBIC INTERVAL: 5 minutes
- **Bike** at 50+ RPMs with moderate tension **OR**
- **Walk** on a slight incline at 2.7 MPH **OR**
- **Use an elliptical trainer or stepper** with moderate resistance

5. MARCH IN PLACE ON TOES: 50 reps
Rest the aerobic bar across your shoulders with feet shoulder-width apart. Lift your left knee straight up at least waist high. Keep your back straight and abdominals contracted. Lower left foot to start-

ing position, keeping on toes at all times. Repeat up-and-down motion with your right knee to complete one rep.

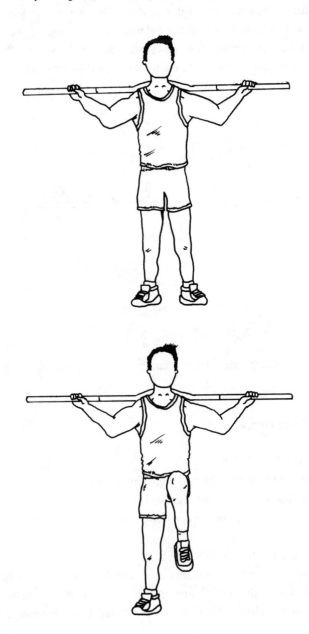

6. SIDE BENDERS: 15 to 20 reps

Rest the aerobic bar across your shoulders. Bend sideways at the waist to the right, and then the left to complete one rep. Keep your lower body still with feet shoulder-width apart.

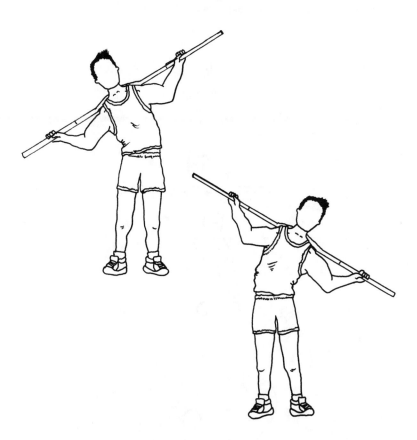

7. DEAD LIFTS: 10 to 15 reps

Grip the weight bar with hands shoulder-width apart, palms down. With arms fully extended, rest the bar lightly on your thighs. Keep your elbows at your sides, your feet 6 inches apart and your knees slightly bent. Inhale as you bend at the hips, lowering the bar as far as you can, almost brushing the front of your legs on the way down. *Back is straight from the hips up!* Exhale as you straighten to the start position. Keep arms fully extended, back straight and the bar close to your body. As you become more accomplished at this exercise, try squeezing your buttocks as you straighten up. Please note: If you have tight hamstrings or lower back pain, be careful with this exercise.

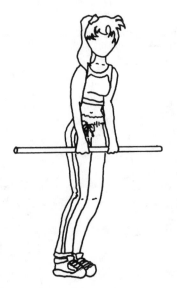

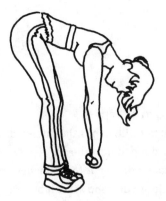

8. UPPER-BODY ROUTINE: 15 reps for all exercises

- **Push-outs:** Keep your back straight, knees slightly flexed and feet shoulder-width apart. Grip aerobic bar, palms facing down, just wider than shoulder-width apart. Raise bar up just above your chest line with elbows up and wrists firm. Extend arms straight out, holding bar above chest level as you exhale. Keeping arms straight, lower bar to the front of your thighs. Inhale while you raise your arms for the next rep, exhale as you push out. Keep entire body aligned and still.

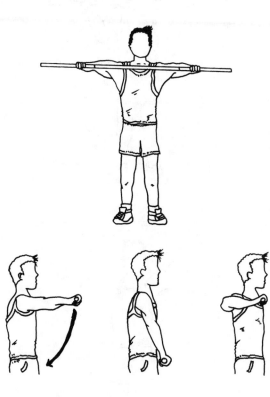

- **Behind-the-Neck Press:** Keep back straight, knees flexed and feet shoulder-width apart. Grip aerobic bar with palms facing outward just wider than shoulder-width apart and rest it lightly on your shoulders behind your neck. Extend your arms straight up while exhaling. Now bend your arms, lowering the bar to the start position as you inhale.

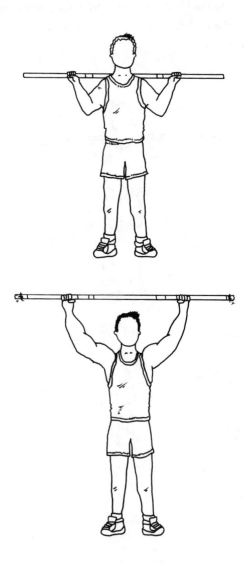

- **Front Press:** Keep back straight, knees flexed and feet shoulder-width apart. Grip aerobic bar with palms facing outward just wider than shoulder-width apart and rest bar across top of chest. Extend your arms, raising the bar straight up while you exhale. Bend your arms and slowly return bar to the start position as you inhale.

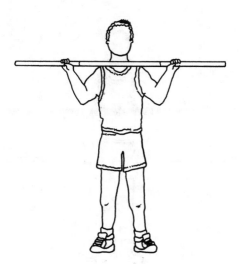

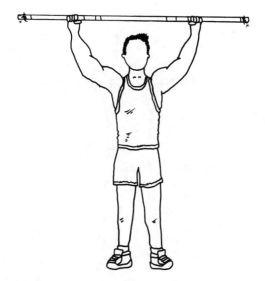

- **Upright Rows:** Keep back straight, knees flexed and feet shoulder-width apart. Grip aerobic bar, palms facing down, hands 6 to 12 inches apart. Hold bar with arms fully extended against the front of your thighs. Slowly raise bar toward your chin, keeping elbows above bar level as you exhale. Return to the start position as you inhale.

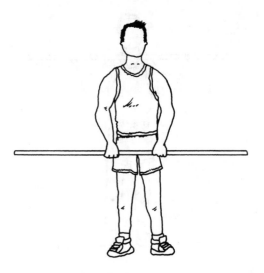

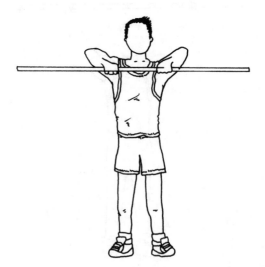

- **Bicep Curl:** Keep back straight, knees flexed and feet shoulder-width apart. Grip aerobic bar, palms facing up, hands shoulder-width apart. Hold bar with arms fully extended against the front of your thighs. Keeping wrists firm and elbows at your side, curl the bar up to your chest as you exhale. Slowly return bar to the start position as you inhale.

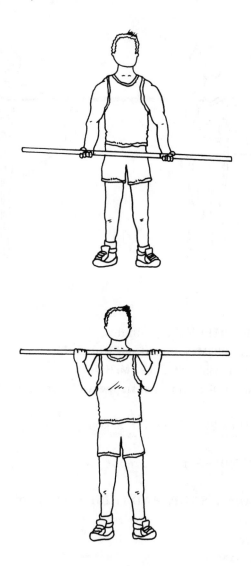

- **Tricep Kickbacks:** Keep back straight, knees flexed and feet shoulder-width apart. Grip aerobic bar behind your back. Start with the bar resting lightly against the buttocks, palms facing outward. Keeping elbows and wrists firm, raise the bar up and back as you exhale. Keeping arms straight, lower bar to the start position as you inhale.

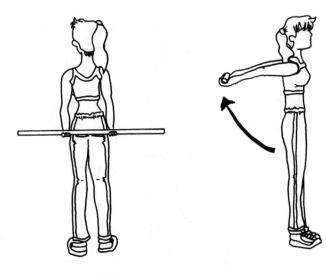

9. **AEROBIC INTERVAL:** 5 minutes
   - **Bike** at 50+ RPMs with moderate tension **OR**
   - **Walk** on a slight incline at 2.7 MPH **OR**
   - **Use an elliptical trainer or stepper** with moderate resistance

10. **MARCH IN PLACE ON TOES:** 50 reps

11. **SIDE BENDERS:** 15 to 20 reps

12. **ABDOMINALS, HIPS AND THIGHS:** 20 reps of each
    - Sit-ups
    - Leg-outs
    - Elbows to Knees

- Knees to Elbows
- Sit-ups (again!)

13. DEAD LIFTS: 10 to 15 reps

14. COOLDOWN: 2 to 3 minutes
- **Bike** leisurely *OR*
- **Walk,** then stretch hamstrings

BEGINNER OFF-DAY ROUTINE

This off-day routine is to be performed in conjunction with your body-type workout. It is designed for those who are seeking to lose weight and/or add additional workouts to their exercise regime. I advise you to perform 2 or 3 off-day routines per week until you've slimmed down to your ideal weight, then cut back to 1 or 2 days per week thereafter. This routine should take approximately 45 minutes to complete. All exercises are illustrated in the beginner core workout.

1. WARM-UP: 30 minutes
- **Bike** at 60+ RPMs at moderate tension *OR*
- **Walk** on a slight incline at 2.7 MPH *OR*
- **Use an elliptical trainer or stepper** with moderate resistance

2. STRETCH: 2 to 4 minutes. Perform each stretch for 30 to 60 seconds.
- Arm Circles
- Triceps
- Upper Back and Chest Stretch
- Spine Twist
- Hamstrings
- Legs-Apart Hamstrings
- Groin
- Quadriceps
- Calves

3. ABDOMINALS, HIPS AND THIGHS: 20 reps for each

- Sit-ups
- Leg-outs
- Elbows to Knees
- Knees to Elbows

4. PUSH-UPS: 5 reps, rest for 30 seconds, then repeat

Start on hands and knees, your body a straight line from your shoulders to your knees, with your ankles crossed. Hands slightly wider than shoulder-width apart, fingers pointing forward and abdominals should be contracted. Inhale as you lower your chest as close to the floor as possible. Exhale as you push yourself up to the starting position. Don't lock your elbows.

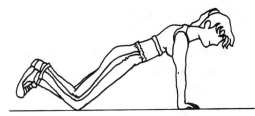

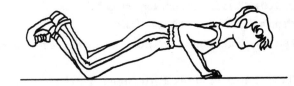

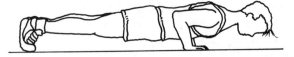

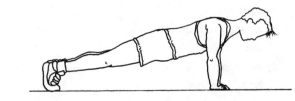

5. **COOLDOWN:** 2 to 3 minutes
   - **Bike** leisurely *OR*
   - **Walk,** then stretch hamstrings

ACTIVE CORE WORKOUT

This workout should be done 3 times per week, with each session lasting approximately 50 minutes. All exercises are illustrated in the beginner core workout.

1. **WARM-UP:** 10 to 20 minutes
   - **Bike** at 70 + RPMs with moderate to high tension *OR*
   - **Jog** (with or without treadmill) on a slight incline at 5.0 + MPH *OR*
   - **Use an elliptical trainer or stepper** with moderate to high resistance

2. **STRETCH:** 2 to 4 minutes. Perform each stretch for 30 to 60 seconds.
   - Arm Circles
   - Triceps
   - Upper Back and Chest Stretch
   - Spine Twist
   - Hamstrings
   - Legs-Apart Hamstrings
   - Groin
   - Quadriceps
   - Calves

3. **ABDOMINALS, HIPS AND THIGHS:** 40 reps each
   - Sit-ups
   - Leg-outs
   - Elbows to Knees
   - Knees to Elbows

4. **AEROBIC INTERVAL:** 5 minutes
   - **Bike** at 70+ RPMs with moderate to high tension *OR*
   - **Jog** (with or without treadmill) on a slight incline at 5.0 + MPH *OR*
   - **Use an elliptical trainer or stepper** with moderate to high resistance

5. MARCH IN PLACE ON TOES: 75 reps

6. SIDE BENDERS: 1 minute

7. DEAD LIFTS: 25 to 35 reps

8. UPPER-BODY ROUTINE: 25 reps of each
- Push-outs
- Behind-the-Neck Press
- Front Press
- Upright Rows
- Bicep Curls
- Tricep Kickbacks

9. AEROBIC INTERVAL: 5 minutes
- **Bike** at 70+ RPMs with moderate to high tension **OR**
- **Jog** (with or without treadmill) on a slight incline at 5.0+ MPH **OR**
- **Use an elliptical trainer or stepper** with moderate to high resistance

10. MARCH IN PLACE: 75 reps

11. SIDE BENDERS: 1 minute

12. ABDOMINALS, HIPS AND THIGHS: 25 reps of each
- Sit-ups
- Leg-outs
- Elbows to Knees
- Knees to Elbows

13. DEAD LIFTS: 25 to 35 reps

14. COOLDOWN: 2 to 3 minutes
- **Bike** leisurely **OR**
- **Walk,** then stretch hamstrings

ACTIVE OFF-DAY ROUTINE

This off-day routine is to be performed in conjunction with your body-type workout. It is designed for those who are seeking to lose weight and/or add additional workouts to their exercise regime. I advise you to perform 2 or 3 off-day routines per week until you've slimmed down to your ideal weight, then ease up and go to 1 or 2 days per week thereafter. This routine should take approximately 45 minutes to complete. All exercises are illustrated in the beginner core workout.

1. **WARM-UP:** 30 minutes
   - **Bike** at 80+ RPMs at moderate to high tension *OR*
   - **Jog** on a slight incline at 5.0 MPH *OR*
   - **Use an elliptical trainer or stepper** with moderate to high tension

2. **STRETCH:** 2 to 4 minutes. Perform each stretch for 30 to 60 seconds.
   - Arm Circles
   - Triceps
   - Upper Back and Chest Stretch
   - Spine Twist
   - Hamstrings
   - Legs-Apart Hamstrings
   - Groin
   - Quadriceps
   - Calves

3. **ABDOMINALS, HIPS AND THIGHS:** 40 reps of each
   - Sit-ups
   - Leg-outs
   - Elbows to Knees
   - Knees to Elbows

4. **PUSH-UPS:** 15 reps

5. **AEROBIC INTERVAL:** 5 to 10 minutes
   - **Jump rope,** *alternating with* 1 minute of side benders as needed to catch your breath *OR*
   - **Favorite aerobic piece**

6. **COOLDOWN:** 2 to 3 minutes
   - **Bike** leisurely *OR*
   - **Walk,** then stretch hamstrings

ADVANCED CORE WORKOUT

This workout should be done 3 times per week, with each session lasting approximately 60 minutes. All exercises are illustrated in the beginner core workout.

1. **WARM-UP:** 10 to 20 minutes
   - **Bike** at 90+ RPMs with high tension **OR**
   - **Run** (with or without treadmil) on a steep incline at 6.0 MPH **OR**
   - **Use an elliptical trainer or stepper** with high resistance

2. **STRETCH:** 2 to 4 minutes. Perform each stretch for 30 to 60 seconds.
   - Arm Circles
   - Triceps
   - Upper Back and Chest Stretch
   - Spine Twist
   - Hamstrings
   - Legs-Apart Hamstrings
   - Groin
   - Quadriceps
   - Calves

3. **ABDOMINALS, HIPS AND THIGHS:** 60 reps of each
   - Sit-ups
   - Leg-outs
   - Elbows to Knees
   - Knees to Elbows

4. **AEROBIC INTERVAL:** 5 minutes
   - **Bike** at 90+ RPMs with high tension **OR**
   - **Run** (with or without treadmill) on a steep incline at 6.0 MPH **OR**
   - **Use an elliptical trainer or stepper** with high resistance

5. **MARCH IN PLACE ON TOES:** 100 reps

6. SIDE BENDERS: 1 minute

7. DEAD LIFTS: 50 reps

8. UPPER-BODY ROUTINE: 40 to 50 reps of each
- Push-outs
- Behind-the-Neck Press
- Front Press
- Upright Rows
- Bicep Curls
- Tricep Kickbacks

9. AEROBIC INTERVAL: 5 minutes
- **Bike** at 90+ RPMs with high tension **OR**
- **Run** (with or without treadmill) on steep incline at 6.0 MPH **OR**
- **Use an elliptical trainer or stepper** with high resistance

10. MARCH IN PLACE ON TOES: 100 reps

11. SIDE BENDERS: 1 minute

12. ABDOMINALS, HIPS AND THIGHS: 60 reps of each

13. DEAD LIFTS: 50 reps

14. COOLDOWN: 2 to 3 minutes
- **Bike** leisurely **OR**
- **Walk,** then stretch hamstrings

ADVANCED OFF-DAY ROUTINE

This off-day routine is to be performed in conjunction with your body-type workout. It is designed for those who are seeking to lose weight and/or add additional workouts to their exercise regime. I advise you to perform 2 or 3 off-day routines per week until you've slimmed down to your ideal weight, then ease up and go to 1 or 2 days per week thereafter. This routine should take approximately 45 minutes to complete. All exercises are illustrated in the beginner core workout.

1. **WARM-UP:** 30 minutes
   - **Bike** at 100+ RPMs with high tension *OR*
   - **Run** with a steep incline at 6.0 MPH *OR*
   - **Use an elliptical trainer or stepper** with high resistance

2. **STRETCH:** 2 to 4 minutes. Perform each stretch for 30 to 60 seconds.
   - Arm Circles
   - Triceps
   - Upper Back and Chest Stretch
   - Spine Twist
   - Hamstrings
   - Legs-Apart Hamstrings
   - Groin
   - Quadriceps
   - Calves

3. **ABDOMINALS, HIPS AND THIGHS:** 60 reps of each
   - Sit-ups
   - Leg-outs
   - Elbows to Knees
   - Knees to Elbows

4. **PUSH-UPS:** 25 reps, rest for 30 seconds, repeat 25 reps

5. **AEROBIC INTERVAL:** 5 to 10 minutes
   - **Jump rope,** *alternating with* 1-minute intervals of side benders as needed to catch your breath

6. **COOLDOWN:** 2 to 3 minutes
   - **Bike** leisurely *OR*
   - **Walk,** then stretch hamstrings

MOVING FORWARD

If you're trying to lose weight, concentrate your efforts on extending the amount of time you can jump rope continuously. Build toward jumping rope for the entire 5-minute aerobic intervals instead of biking, walking, jogging or using the elliptical trainer or stepper. Eventually you want to collapse several 5-minute intervals into one monster 20-minute interval. If you stick to a consistent workout schedule and keep challenging yourself as you become more and more fit, you should be able to reach that goal in about 3 months.

I recommend this approach only to overweight Rulers because if you are not overweight, jumping rope may result in more mass and weight loss than you intend. If you cannot jump rope because of a medical or orthopedic concern and your goal is to shed some pounds, perform as many off-day routines as you can using any piece of aerobic equipment that is safe for your condition. Typically, if you cannot jump rope, you can't run either, so I recommend you rely on a recumbent bike to meet your aerobic-workout needs.

On the anaerobic front, you want to work up to 60 to 100 repetitions of all your abdominal exercises. You should be able to do 50 reps of each upper-body exercise before you make the switch from the lighter bar to a heavier, more challenging weight bar.

If you are considerably overweight, you should ease up on the push-ups or eliminate them altogether until you have shed some weight. Similarly, ease up on the resistance/tension for all of your lower-body aerobic and anaerobic exercises. Don't skip any of the exercises unless a medical or orthopedic condition prevents you from doing so. Even if you initially can perform only very few repetitions of a particular exercise at the start, don't worry, within a very short time you will master it and be ready for more!

CHAPTER 10

The Cone Workout

Welcome, Cones. Your goal is to trim your upper body, specifically your chest, back, upper arms and midsection. As you slim down in these areas, shrinking the gap between your shirt size and your skirt or pants size, your body will appear better proportioned. Because of the excess weight up top, Cones are more susceptible to certain health risks than any of the other 3 body types. Male Cones should shift their focus from the size and strength of their upper bodies to concentrate instead on building muscle in their legs to balance upper- and lower-body strength.

All Cones should earmark 3 days a week for their core workouts. Those who are overweight should supplement with additional 2 to 3 days of off-day routines. Try doing your core workout on Mondays, Wednesdays and Fridays and your off-day routine on the days in between. Allow yourself a one-day break between core workouts. It's okay to perform back-to-back off-day routines because they're less physically demanding.

TOOLS NEEDED
Women

- Stationary bike, treadmill, elliptical or stepper*
- 4-pound aerobic bar
- Exercise mat
- Jump rope

Men

- Stationary bike, treadmill, elliptical or stepper*
- 4-pound aerobic bar
- 10-pound curl bar
- Exercise mat
- Jump rope

* PLEASE NOTE: IF YOU DO NOT HAVE ACCESS TO A STATIONARY BIKE OR A TREADMILL, YOU CAN WALK OR MARCH IN PLACE FOR THE AEROBIC PORTIONS OF YOUR WORKOUT (OR SEE BODY TYPE AND AEROBIC FITNESS EQUIPMENT CHART, PAGE 50).

AEROBIC AND ANAEROBIC INTERVALS

Cones, especially overweight ones, need to improve their posture and hamstring flexibility by strengthening their abdominals and lower backs. During your upper-body anaerobic work, be sure to use only the lowest resistance/tension settings. You'll want to do just the reverse for your lower-body anaerobic work—use the highest resistance and tension settings—provided that you are not overweight. To get rid of a bulging stomach and to decrease the size of your arms, chest and back, it's important to devote at least half your workout to aerobic exercise. A light speed jump rope is the most effective tool for trimming upper arms, back and stomach. Jumping rope will trim your lower body, too, so you may need to use higher-resistance settings on all other lower-body exercises—both aerobic and anaerobic—so that your body balances out. Once you've reached your scale-weight goal, you can split your workout evenly between aerobic and anaerobic exercises, giving special attention to your midsection.

INCREASING YOUR INTENSITY

As a Cone, raising your intensity for lower-body exercises is straightforward. There are a number of ways to rev it up down below. You can increase your speed whether you're jogging, biking or using an elliptical trainer or stepper. You can increase the resistance settings for *all* lower-body exercises (provided, of course, you're not overweight, in which case you should adjust your speed). As your conditioning improves, you can increase both speed and resistance at the same time.

Things get a little more complicated when it comes to your upper body. If you are a very large Cone (in size, not necessarily weight), you may have to stick to high repetitions with very light resistance for the rest of your exercise life. To increase intensity, you want to build up to as many repetitions as possible, taking fewer and fewer breaks as you increase your fitness level. You'll reap both aerobic and anaerobic benefits. This approach will tone and trim you at the same time. Jumping rope at very high RPMs with a light speed rope will intensify your workout and you'll reach your goals faster. Working through your abdominals with as few breaks as possible ensures that you will maximize their calorie-burning power.

Please note: Cone workouts are patent pending.

BEGINNER CORE WORKOUT

The beginner core workout should be done 3 times per week, with each session lasting approximately 40 to 50 minutes.

1. **WARM-UP:** 10 to 20 minutes
   - **Bike** at 50+RPMs with moderate tension **OR**
   - **Walk** (with or without treadmill) using slight incline at 2.5+ MPH **OR**
   - **Use an elliptical trainer or stepper** with moderate resistance

2. STRETCH: 2 to 4 minutes. Perform each stretch for 30 to 60 seconds.

- **Arm Circles:** Stand up straight, knees slightly flexed, feet shoulder-width apart. With arms outstretched, slowly circle your arms forward for 5 revolutions. Make as large a circle as you can. Then reverse and circle your arms backward for 5 revolutions.

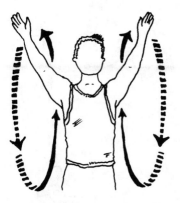

- **Triceps:** With arms straight overhead, bend your right arm so that your right elbow is behind your head. Place your left palm on your right elbow and gently press that elbow toward the wall behind you until you feel the stretch in your shoulder and triceps. Switch arms and repeat.

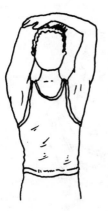

- **Upper Back and Chest Stretch:** Bend forward at the waist, with knees slightly bent. Grasp your hands behind your back, then lift your arms up and hold until you feel a good stretch in your chest, and in the front of your shoulders and upper arms.

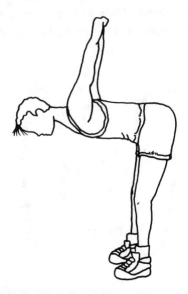

- **Spine Twist:** Sit with both legs extended straight in front of you. Cross your right leg over your left, placing your right foot flat on the floor to the left of your left knee. Turn your upper body clockwise (to the right) and place your right hand palm down on the floor be-

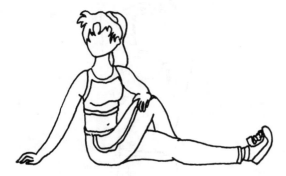

hind you. With your left elbow or hand pressing against the out-side of your right knee, turn your torso as far to the right (clock-wise) as you can as you look over your right shoulder. Reverse arms and legs, twisting your torso to the left (counterclockwise).

- **Hamstrings:** Sit with your legs extended straight in front of you. Bend forward from the hips and reach for your toes. If you can, grab your toes and hold.

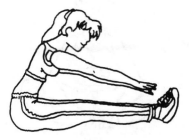

- **Legs-Apart Hamstrings:** Sit with your legs extended and spread as far apart as you can. Bend forward at the hips, moving your hands toward your ankles. Grab your ankles (or the top of your shoes, if you can), gently pull your upper body forward and hold.

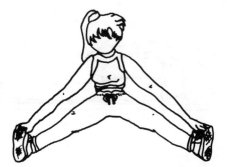

- **Groin:** In a seated position, bring the soles of your shoes together and hold them in place by grabbing your ankles. Gently pull your heels toward your groin. Let your knees relax toward the mat, then press your elbows down on your knees to increase the stretch. Hold when you feel the stretch in your inner thigh and groin.

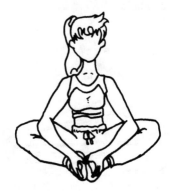

- **Quadriceps:** Lie down on your right side. Bend your left leg back and grab your left ankle with your left hand. Gently pull your leg back toward your buttocks. Hold when you feel a comfortable stretch in the front of your thigh. Release and roll over onto your left side and repeat.

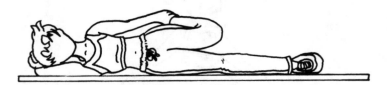

- **Calves:** Stand with your right leg forward and bent at the knee, your left leg fully extended behind you. Place both hands palms flat up against a wall and lean forward. Think about pressing your left heel into the floor. Hold. Then switch legs and repeat.

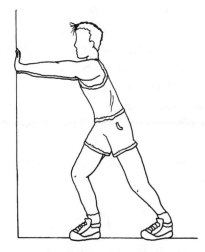

- **Calves (Alternative):** Get down on all fours. Straighten your legs, keeping your palms flat on the floor in front of you. Press your right heel down toward the floor while your left heel is off the floor, left toe touching the floor. After stretching the right calf, switch foot positions so that you are now pressing the heel of your left foot toward the floor while your right heel is off the floor.

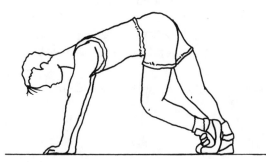

3. AEROBIC INTERVAL: 5 minutes

- **Bike** at 50 + RPMs with moderate tension **OR**
- **Walk** (with or without treadmill) on a slight incline at 2.5+ MPH **OR**
- **Use an elliptical trainer or stepper** with moderate resistance

4. UPPER-BODY ROUTINE (with a 4-pound aerobic bar for women or a 10-pound curl bar for men): 20 reps of each

- **Push-outs:** Keep your back straight, knees slightly flexed and feet shoulder-width apart. Grip aerobic bar, palms facing down, just wider than shoulder-width apart. Raise bar up just above your chest line with elbows up and wrists firm. Extend arms straight out, holding bar above chest level as you exhale. Keeping arms straight, lower bar to the front of your thighs. Inhale while you raise your arms for the next rep, exhale as you push out. Keep entire body aligned and still.

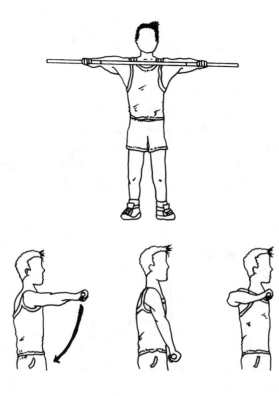

- **Behind-the-Neck Press:** Keep back straight, knees flexed and feet shoulder-width apart. Grip aerobic bar with palms facing outward just wider than shoulder-width apart and rest it lightly on your shoulders behind your neck. Extend your arms straight up while exhaling. Now bend your arms, lowering the bar to the start position as you inhale.

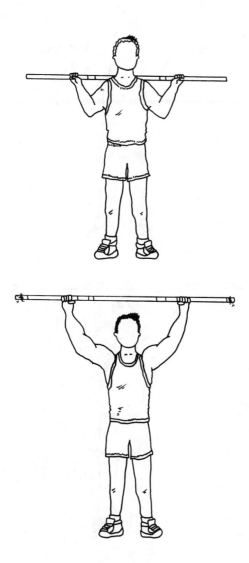

- **Front Press:** Keep back straight, knees flexed and feet shoulder-width apart. Grip aerobic bar with palms facing outward just wider than shoulder-width apart and rest bar across top of chest. Extend your arms, raising the bar straight up while you exhale. Bend your arms and slowly return bar to the start position as you inhale.

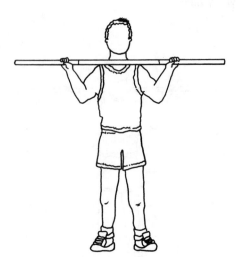

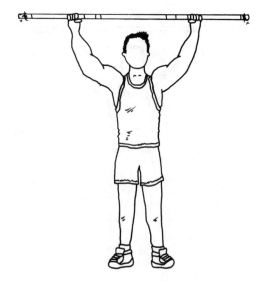

- **Upright Rows:** Keep back straight, knees flexed and feet shoulder-width apart. Grip aerobic bar, palms facing down, hands 6 to 12 inches apart. Hold bar with arms fully extended against the front of your thighs. Slowly raise bar toward your chin, keeping elbows above bar level as you exhale. Return to the start position as you inhale.

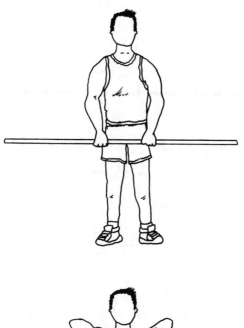

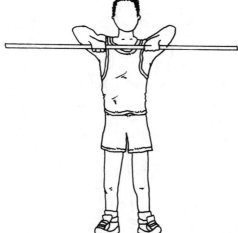

- **Bicep Curl:** Keep back straight, knees flexed and feet shoulder-width apart. Grip aerobic bar, palms facing up, hands shoulder-width apart. Hold bar with arms fully extended against the front of your thighs. Keeping wrists firm and elbows at your side, curl the bar up to your chest as you exhale. Slowly return bar to the start position as you inhale.

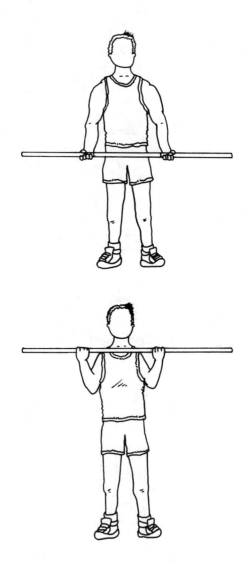

- **Tricep Kickbacks:** Keep back straight, knees flexed and feet shoulder-width apart. Grip aerobic bar behind your back. Start with the bar resting lightly against the buttocks, palms facing outward. Keeping elbows and wrists firm, raise the bar up and back as you exhale. Keeping arms straight, lower bar to the start position as you inhale.

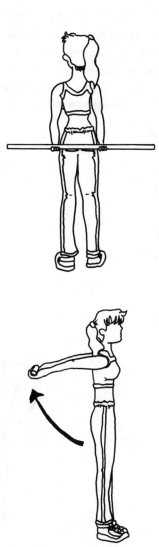

5. DEAD LIFTS: 10 to 20 reps

Grip the weight bar with hands shoulder-width apart, palms down. With arms fully extended, rest the bar lightly on your thighs. Keep your elbows at your sides, your feet 6 inches apart and your knees slightly bent. Inhale as you bend at the hips, lowering the bar as far as you can, almost brushing the front of your legs on the way down. *Back is straight from the hips up!* Exhale as you straighten to the start position. Keep arms fully extended, back straight and the bar close to your body. As you become more accomplished at this exercise, try squeezing your buttocks as you straighten up. Please note: If you have tight hamstrings or lower back pain, be careful with this exercise.

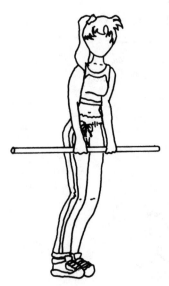

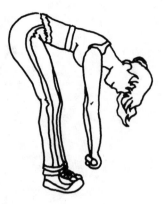

6. SIDE BENDERS: 25 to 50 reps

Rest the aerobic bar across your shoulders. Bend sideways at the waist to the right, and then the left to complete one rep. Keep your lower body still with your feet shoulder-width apart.

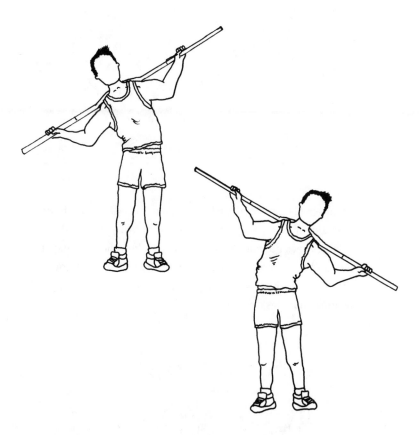

7. ABDOMINALS, HIPS AND THIGHS: 20 reps for all exercises

- **Sit-ups:** Lie on your back with knees bent, feet flat on the floor, fingertips at your temples. Slowly raise your head and shoulders off the ground until your elbows touch your knees as you exhale. Lower to the starting position and inhale. For an easier sit-up, perform with arms fully extended, as shown below.

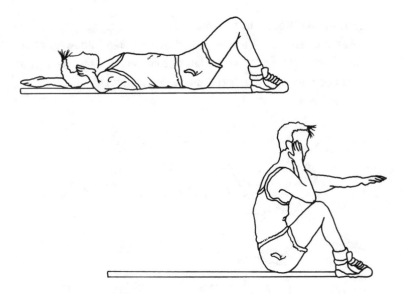

- **Leg-outs:** Lie on your back, with hands under your buttocks, palms down, and bring both knees in toward your chest. Slowly straighten legs out with toes pointed. Inhale while bringing knees toward chest, exhale as you straighten your legs. Beginners can raise their legs higher, but as your abdominals grow stronger, try lowering your legs closer to the mat.

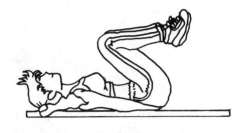

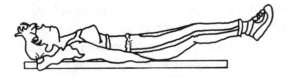

- **Elbows to Knees:** Lie on your back. Raise knees and feet toward your chest. Clasp your hands together at the base of your neck, then curl your upper body, bringing your elbows to your knees. Slowly lower your upper body to the mat. The lower half of your body remains motionless. Exhale as you bring elbows to knees.

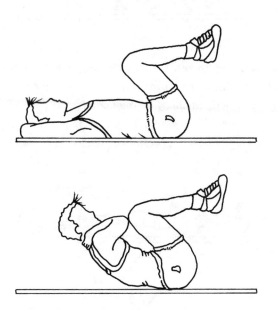

- **Knees to Elbows:** Lie on the floor, with hands clasped at the base of your neck. Raise your head and shoulders off the floor. Your upper body remains in this position. Now raise your knees and feet in a tucked position toward your elbows, keeping your lower back pressed to the floor. Lower your toes to the ground, then exhale as you raise knees to elbows to begin the next rep.

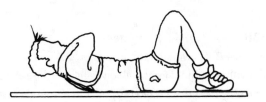

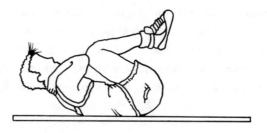

- **Alternate Leg Raises:** Lie on your back with your hands under your buttocks, palms down. Raise your right leg to a 90-degree angle, your left remaining on the floor. Pressing the small of your back into the floor, lower your right leg as you simultaneously lift your left leg. Repeat this continuous scissoring motion.

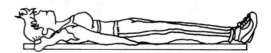

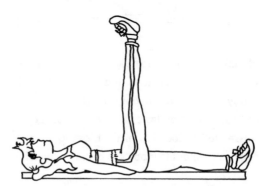

8. **AEROBIC INTERVAL:** 5 minutes
   - **Bike** at 50+ RPMs with moderate tension **OR**
   - **Walk** (with or without treadmill) on a slight incline at 2.5+ MPH **OR**
   - **Use an elliptical trainer or stepper** with moderate resistance

9. MARCH IN PLACE ON TOES: 25 reps

Rest the aerobic bar across your shoulders with feet shoulder-width apart. Lift your left knee straight up at least waist high. Keep your back straight and abdominals contracted. Lower left foot to starting position, keeping on toes at all times. Repeat up-and-down motion with your right knee to complete one rep.

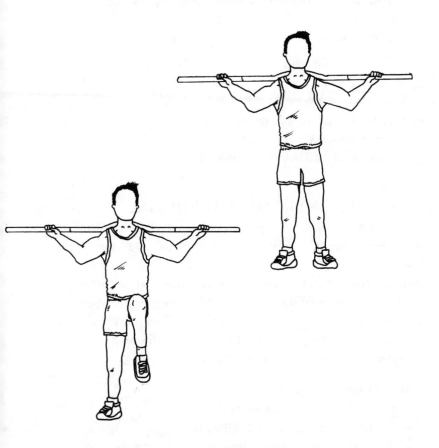

10. UPPER-BODY ROUTINE (with a 4-pound aerobic bar for women or a 10-pound curl bar for men): 20 reps of each

- Push-outs
- Behind-the-Neck Press
- Front Press

- Upright Rows
- Bicep Curls
- Tricep Kickbacks

11. MARCH IN PLACE ON TOES: 25 reps

12. ABDOMINALS, HIPS AND THIGHS: 20 reps each
- Sit-ups
- Elbows to Knees
- Knees to Elbows

13. SIDE BENDERS: 25 to 50 reps

14. COOLDOWN: 2 to 3 minutes
- **Bike** leisurely *OR*
- **Walk**, stretching hamstrings as necessary

BEGINNER OFF-DAY ROUTINE

This off-day routine is to be performed in conjunction with your body-type workout. It is designed for those who are seeking to lose weight and/or add additional workouts to their exercise regime. I advise you to perform 2 or 3 off-day routines per week until you've slimmed down to your ideal weight, then ease up and go to 1 or 2 days per week thereafter. This routine should take approximately 40 minutes to complete. All exercises are illustrated in the beginner core workout.

1. WARM-UP: 30 minutes
- **Bike** at 60+ RPMs with moderate tension *OR*
- **Walk** on a slight incline at 2.7+ MPH *OR*
- **Use an elliptical trainer or stepper** with moderate resistance

2. STRETCH: 2 to 4 minutes. Perform each stretch for 30 to 60 seconds.
- Arm Circles
- Triceps

- Upper Back and Chest Stretch
- Spine Twist
- Hamstrings
- Legs-Apart Hamstrings
- Groin
- Quadriceps
- Calves

3. ABDOMINALS, HIPS AND THIGHS: 20 reps of each
- Sit-ups
- Leg-outs
- Elbows to Knees
- Knees to Elbows

4. SQUAT THRUSTS: 10 reps
Stand with back straight, knees slightly bent and feet shoulder-width apart. Tuck into a squat position, thighs parallel to the mat, palms face down 6 inches in front of your toes and slightly wider than shoulder-width apart. Exhale as you kick both legs out behind you, landing on your toes with legs fully extended. Thrust back into tuck position, then stand up, returning to the start position.

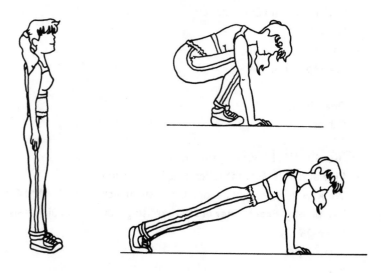

5. SIDE BENDERS: 1 minute

6. COOLDOWN: 2 to 3 minutes
- **Bike** leisurely *OR*
- **Walk,** stretching hamstrings as necessary

ACTIVE CORE WORKOUT

This workout should be done 3 times per week, with each session lasting approximately 60 minutes. All exercises are illustrated in the beginner core workout.

1. WARM-UP: 10 to 20 minutes
- **Bike** at 70+ RPMs with moderate to high tension *OR*
- **Walk** (with or without treadmill) on a slight incline at 3.2+ MPH *OR*
- **Use an elliptical trainer or stepper** using moderate to high resistance

2. STRETCH: 2 to 4 minutes. Perform each stretch for 30 to 60 seconds.
- Arm Circles
- Triceps
- Upper Back and Chest Stretch
- Spine Twist
- Hamstrings
- Legs-Apart Hamstrings
- Groin
- Quadriceps
- Calves

3. AEROBIC INTERVAL: 5 minutes
- **Bike** at 70+ RPMs with moderate to high tension *OR*
- **Walk** (with or without treadmill) on a slight incline at 3.2+ MPH *OR*
- **Use an elliptical trainer or stepper** using moderate to high resistance *OR*
- **Jump rope**

4. **UPPER-BODY ROUTINE** (with a 4-pound aerobic bar for women or a 10-pound weight bar for men): 35 reps of each
   - Push-outs
   - Behind-the-Neck Press
   - Front Press
   - Upright Rows
   - Bicep Curls
   - Tricep Kickbacks

5. **DEAD LIFTS:** 25 reps

6. **SIDE BENDERS:** 1 minute

7. **ABDOMINALS, HIPS AND THIGHS:** 40 reps of each
   - Sit-ups
   - Leg-outs
   - Elbows to Knees
   - Knees to Elbows

8. **AEROBIC INTERVAL:** 5 minutes
   - **Bike** at 70+ RPMs with moderate to high tension *OR*
   - **Walk** (with or without treadmill) on a slight incline at 3.2+ MPH *OR*
   - **Use an elliptical trainer or stepper** with moderate to high resistance *OR*
   - **Jump rope**

9. **MARCH IN PLACE ON TOES:** 50 reps

10. **UPPER-BODY ROUTINE** (with a 4-pound aerobic bar for women or a 10-pound weight bar for men): 35 reps of each
    - Push-outs
    - Behind-the-Neck Press
    - Front Press
    - Upright Rows
    - Bicep Curls
    - Tricep Kickbacks

11. MARCH IN PLACE ON TOES: 50 reps

12. ABDOMINALS, HIPS AND THIGHS: 40 reps of each
- Sit-ups
- Leg-outs
- Elbows to Knees
- Knees to Elbows

13. SIDE BENDERS: 1 minute

14. COOLDOWN: 2 to 3 minutes
- **Bike** leisurely *OR*
- **Walk,** stretching hamstrings as necessary

ACTIVE OFF-DAY ROUTINE

This off-day routine is to be performed in conjunction with your body-type workout. It is designed for those who are seeking to lose weight and/or add additional workouts to their exercise regime. I advise you to perform 2 or 3 off-day routines per week until you've slimmed down to your ideal weight, then ease up and go to 1 or 2 days per week thereafter. This routine should take approximately 45 minutes to complete. All exercises are illustrated in the beginner core workout.

1. WARM-UP: 30 minutes
- **Bike** at 80+ RPMs with moderate tension *OR*
- **Walk** on a slight incline at 3.2 MPH *OR*
- **Use an elliptical trainer or stepper** with moderate to high resistance

2. STRETCH: 2 to 4 minutes. Perform each stretch for 30 to 60 seconds.
- Arm Circles
- Triceps
- Upper Back and Chest Stretch

- Spine Twist
- Hamstrings
- Legs-Apart Hamstrings
- Groin
- Quadriceps
- Calves

3. **ABDOMINALS, HIPS AND THIGHS:** 40 reps of each
   - Sit-ups
   - Leg-outs
   - Elbows to Knees
   - Knees to Elbows

4. **SQUAT THRUSTS:** 20 reps

5. **SIDE BENDERS:** 1 minute

6. **SQUAT THRUSTS:** 20 reps

7. **JUMP ROPE:** 5 minutes

8. **COOLDOWN:** 2 to 3 minutes
   - **Bike** leisurely **OR**
   - **Walk,** stretching hamstrings as necessary

ADVANCED CORE WORKOUT

This workout should be done 3 times per week, with each session lasting approximately 60 minutes. All exercises are illustrated in the beginner core workout.

1. **WARM-UP:** 10 to 20 minutes
   - **Bike** at 100+ RPMs with high tension **OR**
   - **Walk** (with or without treadmill) on a steep incline at 4.0+ MPH **OR**
   - **Use an elliptical trainer or stepper** with high resistance

2. **STRETCH:** 2 to 4 minutes. Perform each stretch for 30 to 60 seconds.
   - Arm Circles
   - Triceps
   - Upper Back and Chest Stretch
   - Spine Twist
   - Hamstrings
   - Legs-Apart Hamstrings
   - Groin
   - Quadriceps
   - Calves

3. **AEROBIC INTERVAL:** 5 minutes
   - **Bike** at 100+ RPMs with high tension **OR**
   - **Walk** (with or without treadmill) on a steep incline at 4.0+ MPH **OR**
   - **Use an elliptical trainer or stepper** with high resistance **OR**
   - **Jump rope**

4. **UPPER-BODY ROUTINE** (with a 4-pound aerobic bar for women or 10-pound curl bar for men): 50 reps of each
   - Push-outs
   - Behind-the-Neck Press
   - Front Press
   - Upright Rows
   - Bicep Curls
   - Tricep Kickbacks

5. **DEAD LIFTS:** 50 reps

6. **SIDE BENDERS:** 1 minute

7. **ABDOMINALS, HIPS AND THIGHS:** 50 reps each
   - Sit-ups
   - Leg-outs
   - Elbows to Knees
   - Knees to Elbows

8. **AEROBIC INTERVAL:** 5 minutes
   - **Bike** at 100+ RPMs with high tension **OR**
   - **Walk** (with or without treadmill) on a steep incline at 4.0+ MPH **OR**
   - **Use an elliptical trainer or stepper** with high resistance **OR**
   - **Jump rope**

9. **MARCH IN PLACE ON TOES:** 75 reps

10. **UPPER-BODY ROUTINE** (with a 4-pound aerobic bar for women or a 10-pound curl bar for men): 30 reps each
    - Push-outs
    - Behind-the-Neck Press
    - Front Press
    - Upright Rows
    - Bicep Curls
    - Tricep Kickbacks

11. **MARCH IN PLACE ON TOES:** 75 reps

12. **ABDOMINALS, HIPS AND THIGHS:** 40 reps
    - Sit-ups
    - Leg-outs
    - Elbows to Knees
    - Knees to Elbows

13. **SIDE BENDERS:** 1 minute

14. **COOLDOWN:** 2 to 3 minutes
    - **Bike** leisurely **OR**
    - **Walk,** stretching hamstrings as necessary

ADVANCED OFF-DAY ROUTINE

This off-day routine is to be performed in conjunction with your body-type workout. It is designed for those who are seeking to lose weight and/or add additional workouts to their exercise regime. I advise you to perform 2 or 3 off-day routines per week until you've slimmed down to your ideal weight, then ease up and go to 1 or 2 days per week thereafter. This routine should take approximately 60 minutes to complete. All exercises are illustrated in the beginner core workout.

1. WARM-UP: 30 minutes
   - **Bike** at 100+ RPMs with high tension **OR**
   - **Walk** at 4.2+ MPH on a steep incline **OR**
   - **Use an elliptical trainer or stepper** with high resistance

2. STRETCH: 2 to 4 minutes. Perform each stretch for 30 to 60 seconds.
   - Arm Circles
   - Triceps
   - Upper Back and Chest Stretch
   - Spine Twist
   - Hamstrings
   - Legs-Apart Hamstrings
   - Groin
   - Quadriceps
   - Calves

3. AEROBIC INTERVAL: 10 minutes
   - **Jump rope OR**
   - **Other favorite aerobic activity**

4. ABDOMINALS, HIPS AND THIGHS: 50 reps
   - Sit-ups
   - Leg-outs
   - Elbows to Knees
   - Knees to Elbows

5. SQUAT THRUSTS: 30 reps

6. SIDE BENDERS: 1 minute

7. SQUAT THRUSTS: 30 reps

8. AEROBIC INTERVAL: 5 minutes
- **Jump rope *OR***
- **Other favorite aerobic activity**

9. COOLDOWN: 2 to 3 minutes
- **Bike** leisurely *OR*
- **Walk,** stretching hamstrings as necessary.

MOVING FORWARD

As your cardiovascular conditioning and muscular strength and endurance improve, you can jump rope for the entire length of each 5-minute aerobic interval if you desire. I don't recommend you do this unless you are overweight. If you're not, you're better off doing high-resistance/tension aerobic work so that you won't lose too much mass down below. If your legs and butt are especially small compared to your upper body, I suggest you add an extra set or 2 of dead lifts with additional weight within your core workout. If you do decide to jump rope, build to no more than 15-minute intervals, which should take you no more than 90 days. If you can't jump rope because of a medical or orthopedic condition, the next best thing is a recumbent bike with the resistance set anywhere from medium to high. You should establish as your goal 75 to 100 repetitions for all mat and upper-body exercises and dead lifts. Try to build to 50 squat thrusts without a rest. And don't forget to pay special attention to those hamstrings. Spend an extra minute or 2 stretching them. You might even take a yoga class once a week to help ease upper-body tightness if you can schedule the time for it.

## CHAPTER 11

I Escaped My Shape! Testimonials

Over the years, my staff at Exude and I have received and collected thousands of testimonials. Some of those you'll find on the following pages come from clientele we've worked with one-on-one, some are from people who saw an article in a magazine and followed the advice within, some are from people for whom we have designed body-type programs via the telephone and Web with our FASTFITNESS Routine and some are from the readers who followed the advice in my previous book, *Hold It! You're Exercising Wrong.*

What you'll read in just these handful of our many testimonials are individual experiences in the exercisers' own words. Some were kind enough to share their before-and-after photos. You'll find a common theme runs through all the testimonials: that consistently working out appropriately for their body types is what got them to the promised land. That's why I'm sharing their stories with you. You'll see a cross section of ages, fitness levels, genders and physical abilities, of individuals who all have improved their health, fitness levels and shape. It's also important to note that some of these testimonials are current and others go back to other decades, which should give you, the reader, confidence that the material and information within this book are real, not a fad or a gimmick. The results really do speak for themselves, so read on.

JACKIE

Age: 34
Body Type: Bottom-Heavy Ruler
Pounds Lost: 25
Inches Lost: 32
Change in Clothing Size: From a 14 to an 8
Time Elapsed Between Before-and-After
    Measurements: 6 months
Total Time Exercising: 18 months

Workout History: Jackie never really exercised before she came to Exude for help. While she had set weight-loss goals before, disciplined exercise had never been a part of the plan for meeting those goals. She just "wasn't into it."

Testimonial: For me, being thin had always been about losing weight. What the scale said. I think the turning point for me in my experience with Exude was when it became about being fit. As I gained strength and endurance, it became more about how I felt than about my shrinking pants size. Though, hey, that was great, too!

I had lost weight and gained it back before. There wasn't a fad diet I hadn't tried by the time I desperately crawled into Exude that first morning. In the past my mission had always been to find the easiest and fastest way to lose

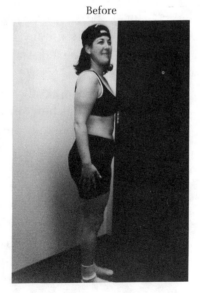

Before

weight. I'm sure that sounds familiar. Exercising and eating sensibly were options that just never occurred to me. Sure, I worked out. I was a member of a nice New York City gym and would "regularly" get there once or twice a week . . . if nothing else came up. I would take high-powered, low-impact "aerobic" classes and be satisfied that I had "exercised." It never dawned on me that the lack of any change in my body (or anyone else's) was a sign that these classes were a waste of my time.

I heard about Edward's program from a wonderful friend of mine. He saw fantastic results in another one of Edward's clients and really pushed me into making the call. I can never thank him enough. After three weeks I felt something I'd never felt before. I began to see unbelievable changes in my body, energy level, and endurance, and most of all, in my self-esteem.

It was different from the way you feel when you are on a great diet and losing weight. You know, people start to notice and say you look thin. This was about the pride and confidence I felt in being able to do something that wasn't easy. I wasn't taking a diet pill and getting skinny. *I was working hard* but *liking it!* I was looking forward to exercising. I knew each workout was bringing me closer to my goal—of being in shape and staying in shape forever.

No more gaining the weight back and then latching on to the next fad diet. On this program, one day of bad eating isn't going to kill me. I know I can maintain control with a balance of exercise and eating. In fact, this is what exercise is supposed to be. It's supposed to burn calories, of course, but also to make you stronger, make you feel and look better.

After

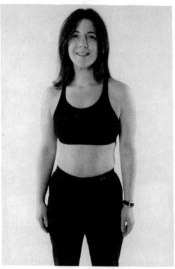

I'm not going to tell you there aren't what I call "those days," those days you don't want to go to the gym, those days the scale shows you've gained a few pounds. We're all human. But this program never, ever fails me. When I get back on track and do my workout, I instantly feel the same sense of pride I felt that first month I began—more than 18 months ago!

Body Part	Before	After	Inches Lost
Chest	40.5	34.5	6
Waist	35	31	4
Hips	43	37	6
Thigh	27	23.5	3.5*
Knee	18.5	16.5	2*
Calf	14	14	0
Tricep	14	11.5	2.5*

* THIS FIGURE REPRESENTS THE INCH LOSS ON ONLY ONE THIGH, KNEE AND ARM.

BEN

Age: 47
Body Type: Cone
Pounds Lost: 135
Inches Lost: 100+
Change in Clothing Size: From 58" to 39" waist
Time Elapsed Between Before-and-After
   Measurements: 18 months
Total Time Exercising: 2 years

Workout History: Ben's doctor referred him to Exude to help him lose weight and lower his blood pressure. His doctor had recommended hip surgery, but wanted him to lose weight first.
Testimonial: Like a lot of other people whose doctors tell them they have high blood pressure (mine was 175/115) and are in

serious danger of other illness because they're overweight (I was just over 350 pounds), I decided to ignore him. After months of "thinking about" his recommendations and pretty much not doing anything to help myself, my doctor suggested that I go to see someone for help—Edward Jackowski. He gave me a copy of Edward's first book, *Hold It! You're Exercising Wrong*.

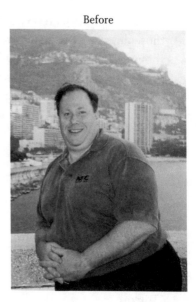

Before

That's when things changed. I read it and met the infectiously enthusiastic man a week later. He recognized my limitations (I hadn't exercised in more than ten years), yet he knew he could help me. We started slowly—in my case at remedial speed. I had to learn to move again. I had finally come to the realization that the only one who was going to make this happen was me (with a lot of help!). Edward devised a program for my body that I could follow, and I did, 4 times a week.

Now it's been 2 years since I began Edward's program and here are the results:

- I've lost 135 pounds.
- My waist has shrunk from a 58 to a 39.
- My suit size is down from a 58 to a 46.
- My resting heart rate is 45.
- My cholesterol is down from 177 to 123.
- My HDL to LDL ratio is 2.4 (down from 6.1), which my doctor says is quite good.
- My severely arthritic hips have both been replaced. My surgeon would never have performed this surgery before I'd lost the weight. I was in so much pain and had such limited range of motion that in the year

prior to surgery, I had to use a cane to walk. After surgery, it took me less than six weeks to progress from walker to crutches to cane to no assistive device at all! Again, pretty good, according to my surgeon. Being in shape *before* the operation really did help.

- My energy level is now *through the roof!* I never thought that I'd actually have more energy by exercising. I'd always thought I should be conserving it.

I honestly feel that Edward Jackowski and his program for my body type helped save my life. Without Edward's program, enthusiasm and support, I doubt that I'd have been able to stick with it. The results I got encouraged me to continue and the results are, in my opinion, due to 2 things: my resolve (you've got to make up your mind to do it) and Edward Jackowski's methodology.

After

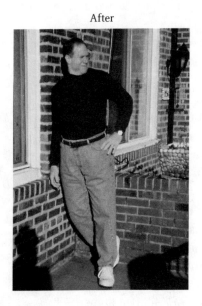

KATHY

Age: 27
Body Type: Hourglass
Pounds Lost: 36
Inches Lost: 30
Change in Clothing Size: From a 10/12 to a 4
Time Elapsed Between Before-and-After Measurements: 6 months
Total Time Exercising: 3 years

Workout History: Kathy used to work out with weights and heavy resistance—disastrous choices that bulked her up and stood in the way of her losing any mass. She started seeing results as soon as she changed her routine to one based on her body type.

Testimonial: In August 1998, I met up with the folks at Exude and was introduced to the Escape Your Shape program. I'd been going to the gym on and off for two years before that. Every time I threw myself into it, I would lose some weight, but I never really changed the way I looked, and I certainly didn't keep the weight off. The harder I worked, the bigger I felt. I didn't have anything to lose with the Escape Your Shape program. After all, I wasn't having much success on my own.

As a working professional, I could spend no more than an hour at the gym at a time. (Let's face it, if we all had three hours a day to devote to exercise and money for

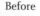
Before

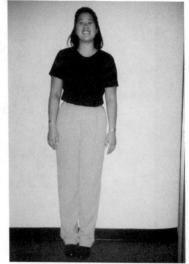

cosmetic alterations, we could all look like movie stars.) I was also traveling for work, so relying on equipment that I might not find in a hotel gym was an issue for me. I made all that clear in my initial interview with the folks at Exude. They designed a program for me based on my body type. It was easy to follow and something I could do at my regular gym, a hotel gym or even in a hotel room. Within the first two weeks I felt and saw a difference. My pants were starting to feel looser. Sure enough, when I weighed myself and measured my problem areas, there were real changes. I was also more energetic. After three months I lost 30 pounds and dropped over three sizes (from a 10/12 to a 4). Friends and family noticed the dramatic changes, too, and more important, I felt better about myself. That affected the rest of my life.

Today, almost three years after I completed the formal program, I still work out along Exude guidelines, though I'm in Hong Kong, halfway around the world from their New York studio. My workouts are a part of my life. When I don't do them, I miss them. I encourage people to try this program. It's easy to follow. I learned which exercises are good for me and how to make the most of my time at the gym, or wherever I happen to be when I carve out workout time. Escape Your Shape has changed my life and I'm grateful. Not only did it change my physical appearance, it gave me the confidence to try other things as well. People I haven't seen in a long time can't help but say, "Wow, you look great! How did you do it?" I think they expect me to tell them I took some kind of weight-loss pill or something, but I just tell them the

After

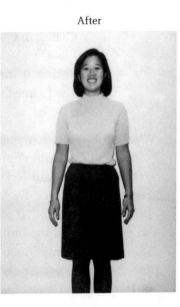

truth. I did it by learning how to exercise right for my body type and lifestyle. Thanks, Exude.

Body Part	Before	After	Inches Lost
Chest	38	33	5
Waist	31	26	5
Hips	39	35	4
Thigh	24	21	3*
Knee	17.5	16	1.5*
Calf	15	14	1*
Tricep	13.5	11	2.5*

* THIS FIGURE REPRESENTS THE INCH LOSS ON ONLY ONE THIGH, KNEE AND ARM.

JANE

Age: 39
Body Type: Top-Heavy Ruler
Pounds Lost: 16+
Inches Lost: 35
Change in Clothing Size: From a 12 to a 6/8
**Time Elapsed Between Before-and-After
    Measurements:** 10 months
Total Time Exercising: 1 year

Workout History: A regular exerciser, Jane was frustrated because her efforts didn't produce results.
Testimonial: Edward Jackowski's exercise program was highly recommended to me by a friend who lost 25 pounds on his program in three months. So while I'm generally a procrastinator, when it came to signing up with Exude, I didn't hesitate for a minute. In fact, my friend's story was so compelling, I signed up for 48 training sessions before I even met Edward.

He promised I would start to see a positive change in my

body in two weeks—even if I made no effort to change my eating habits. I thought it couldn't work. I'd been going to the gym for fifteen years. I was convinced that I was fit and in shape, though I was carrying some extra weight. I exercised three to five times a week with a potpourri of classes from body sculpting, to hip-hop aerobics to power yoga. I gravitated toward the choreographed classes, which improved my coordination and stamina, but didn't burn many calories. So I compensated by running 4 to 5 miles

Before

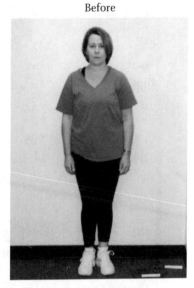

three times a week. My body wasn't happy about that at all. My knees especially. And when I finished, I was so wiped out that I didn't have the energy for floor work. A big mistake! All that activity was good for my coordination, endurance and stamina, but it just wasn't changing my body. In fact, I put on twenty pounds over those fifteen years though I wasn't eating any more.

I am what you would call a full-figured gal (like Jane Russell, for those of you who remember), with hips, breasts, broad shoulders and swimmer's arms. I tend to gain weight on my top half a little faster than down below. Edward subscribes to what I call the "combo platter" of exercise: a little cardio, a little stretching and a little anaerobic activity with exercises on the mat and upper-body exercises with a 4- to 8-pound bar. For the first two or three months every time I would see Edward, I would swear at him. I had a hard time getting used to the jump rope and hated jumping jacks. Then one day it all fell into place.

Edward turned out to be right. Four months after I started, I was like a new person. I'd lost more than 16 pounds and 24

Body Part	Before	After	Inches Lost
Chest	41	36	5
Waist	36	30	6
Hips	40	36	4
Thigh	25.5	22.5	3*
Knee	19	16.5	2.5*
Calf	14.5	13.0	1.5*
Tricep	14.5	11.5	3*

* This figure represents the inch loss on only one thigh, knee and arm.

inches with very few changes to my diet. I was able to slither into one of my favorite night dresses that I'd pushed to the back of my closet into the "reserved for later" section. "Later" had arrived!

One year after working out the Exude way, a great weight has been lifted off me—literally! I've lost 16 pounds and more than 20 inches, a feat I accomplished not by starving myself—my former method of choice—but by exercising the right way for my body type and goals. I'm now 5 pounds from my target weight, and as James Brown said, "I feel good!"

After

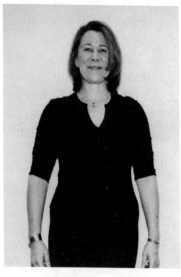

Today, instead of swearing at Edward, I swear by my jump rope. It is, in my opinion, one of the best tools out there for burning calories, and it's fun. You can do it at home, and the better you get at it, the more effective it becomes. It's great for coordination and it fuels your body with oxygen. If you're looking for a way to lose weight, stick with that rope.

One of the most important lessons I've learned from Edward is how to make an hour-long workout work for you. I once exercised regularly, but not in a way that was bringing about change. Now I work out in a way that works for me. Along the way, as I grew stronger, we fine-tuned my routine. Today I work out at a very advanced level and I know that if I stay at this level of fitness and remain consistent and disciplined about my workouts, I won't gain weight. It's nice to set goals for yourself and meet them. It's something you can be proud of.

MICHAEL

Age: 44
Body Type: Ruler
Pounds Lost: 52
Inches Lost: 30+
Change in Clothing Size: 46" to a 38" waist
Time Elapsed Between Before-and-After
    Measurements: 18 months
Total Time Exercising: 2.5 years

Workout History: Michael hadn't worked out regularly since college.

Testimonial: November 9, 1973, was a cool autumn afternoon in Ithaca, New York. I was playing lineman on the Cornell freshman football squad's game against Princeton. Early in the first quarter I landed the wrong way on the Astroturf, which in reality is just a thin shag carpet laid over cement, bearing no resemblance to turf at all. It became immediately apparent that my elbow was dislocated.

Later that evening, after a trip to the emergency room, my roommate and a future doctor, Jon, tried to console me about my season-ending injury. He also saw it as an opportunity to introduce me to the world of sex, drugs and rock and roll. And so began a five-year odyssey of overindulgence. Gone were the

barking coaches. Gone were the
laps around the track. Gone were
regular workouts.

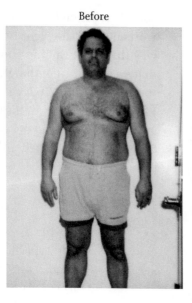

What did remain were my eating habits. The diet of a football
lineman is not exactly what the
Surgeon General prescribes. Jon's
guiding instruction in overindulgence stuck, too. I soon settled into
a pattern of eating, drinking and
little else.

Fast-forward to New Year's Day,
1998. My bride presented me with
the gift of a gym membership.
After listening to me swear for
several long minutes, she took
cover behind the children and pleaded with me to try it. Appar-
ently she cooked up this scheme with a client of mine who also
happened to be an Exude addict. At that point I could only as-
sume that Edward was adding something to the water—à la Jim
Jones—to elicit such devotion.

On February 9, 1998, I found myself dressed in gray sweats
listening to Edward as I attempted my first push-up in 25 years.
The years had not been kind. My memory of the number of sit-
ups, push-ups and even toe touches I could do far exceeded
what I was actually able to do that day on Fifty-second Street.
As I moaned and groaned through the exercises, I began to plan
my escape. Clearly this gym thing was not for me.

At first it seemed like a no-brainer. Listen to the speech, set
up a few appointments, blow them off and let the whole thing
die a slow death. Week One went according to plan. I purchased
new sneakers (a cover-up move) and attended the first scheduled session. I managed to find two good excuses and voilà! By
the end of Week One, I had blown off two of the three sessions.

I forgot that a week has seven days. Sunday morning, as I

was getting a second cup of coffee to go with my second buttered bagel, the doorbell rang. It was Edward. He was on his way to the Hamptons and he thought he would drop by. Since my wife had paid him already, he was going to make sure I got her money's worth. He made me put down the bagel and climb onto one of his (dreaded) blue mats.

My plan was in trouble. There were multiple forces rallying against me. In addition to my wife and client, he had my secretary on his side, scheduling my appointments. Slowly, grudgingly I began to attend more and more sessions. Soon the results were unmistakable.

I began to improve my physical condition. I began to lose weight. People began to notice and I could even see my feet. It got so bad I even bought shoes with laces since I could now touch my toes. And then bad turned a bit worse. I met the nutritionist.

For the very first time I started to watch what I ate. I gave up my daily two-bagel breakfasts. I found moderation and I found guilt. Now when I reach for a candy bar, I think about the sit-ups. Now when I walk by the bakery, I think about jumping rope. At Exude, I have found better health and a better lifestyle. At Exude, I found friendly folks who wanted to help me on my journey to live longer and better. And at Exude, I have found a conscience. A little bit of guilt, a little voice that keeps me on track. Thanks.

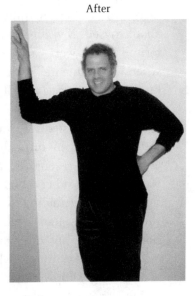

After

MELISSA

Age: 26
Body Type: Hourglass
Pounds Lost: 20
Inches Lost: 27+
Change in Clothing Size: From a 12 to an 8
Time Elapsed Between Before-and-After
 Measurements: 8 months
Total Time Exercising: 2 years

Workout History: Melissa did no regular exercise other than walking before she started the program. Her sister had always been the skinny one. Exercising right for her body type with the right intensity produced results quickly.

Testimonial: I'm writing this to let the world know how drastically my life changed in all but a minute. I spent most of my life dieting or trying anything to take weight off and feel great about myself. My attempts were always successful, but short-term. There were also periods when I experimented with various kinds of exercise—really just dipped my toe in the water. These periods never lasted very long, as I found it extremely difficult to exercise, though I enjoyed the effects on my mind and body. With my weight fluctuating so often, the whole thing took a toll on me both physically and emotionally.

I reached a point where I was feeling simply terrible—my weight reached a place I never wanted it to be. At that very moment, while on a working vaca-

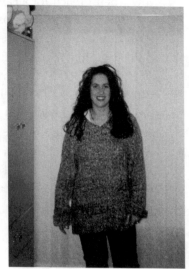

Before

Body Part	Before	After	Inches Lost
Chest	38	36	2
Waist	34.5	29	5.5
Hips	40	37	3
Thigh	25.5	23	2.5*
Knee	18.5	17	1.5*
Calf	16.5	15.5	1*
Tricep	14	10.5	3.5*

* This figure represents the inch loss on only one thigh, knee and arm.

tion, I met Edward Jackowski. From the second we met I sensed his motivational powers. He was overloaded with energy and ready to share it with everyone who encountered him. I'm sure that I was meant to meet this man at that exact moment.

It wasn't long after our meeting that I enrolled in his program at Exude in New York City, where we both live. I chose to work with a personal trainer three times a week for three weeks total. I needed someone to help me stay motivated in one-on-one sessions, as I'm fond of making excuses. My trainer tried to tell me that I'd soon be addicted, that I really didn't need to see him for more than a week. I was sure he was wrong.

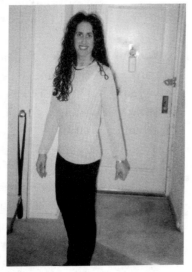

After

He wasn't. Within days I was comfortable with my new routine. Jumping rope proved to be the fastest, most entertaining method of weight loss for my body type. Because I am an Hourglass, my trainer had me do a lot of cardiovascular work *without* a lot of resistance. After a while I found myself looking forward to our sessions and my energy levels soared.

My three weeks came and went quickly. I was officially hooked! I loved how I felt, how I looked and the way everyone noticed the almost immediate results. I continued my routine daily. I didn't need someone else to motivate me. I was doing that for myself. It's been almost two years and I'm still going strong, running 3 to 4 miles every day and jumping rope for half an hour and more. I'm at my ideal weight and feel better than I ever have before. I've never recovered from meeting Edward Jackowski and I hope I never do.

JEN

Age: 33
Body Type: Bottom-Heavy Hourglass
Pounds Lost: 21
Inches Lost: 32+
Change in Clothing Size: From a 14 to an 8
Time Elapsed Between Before-and-After
    Measurements: 9 months
Total Time Exercising: 18 months

Workout History: Jen was an on-again, off-again exerciser for many years. She came to get motivated and lose weight for her wedding, but her workouts didn't stop on her special day.
Testimonial: I am a skeptic—a tough, hardworking New York girl with an attitude. I've been there, done that. No new fitness program was going to solve my weight problem and change my perspective on life—or so I thought.

I had never really enjoyed exercising, nor did I have confidence in my physical abilities. In fact, when I first went to Exude, it had been nearly eight years since I had done any formal or regular exercise. It was October, I was getting married in April and I had to do something fast.

A friend told me about Exude. I was—as usual—not all that

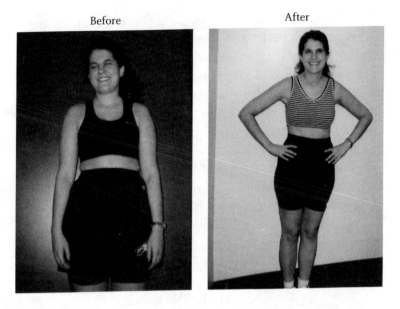

Before   After

interested and was unprepared to make the personal and financial commitments to the program. It was knowing I had to walk down the aisle in the near future that made me take a hard look at my appearance and myself. I was running out of time. I decided to give it a try.

The benefits were amazing. I slowly became a believer in the exercising-for-your-body type. I came to understand how certain

Body Part	Before	After	Inches Lost
Chest	36.5	34	2.5
Waist	32	27	5
Hips	41.5	37.5	4
Thigh	27	23	4*
Knee	19	16.5	2.5*
Calf	16	15	1*
Tricep	14	11	3*

* THIS FIGURE REPRESENTS THE INCH LOSS ON ONLY ONE THIGH, KNEE AND ARM.

kinds of exercise helped me drop inches off certain body parts. The way my clothes fit started to change, and so did my commitment to the right exercise and a lifestyle that included fitness.

There are no magic pills. Edward's formula is simple. Believe in yourself, work hard at exercise, eat right, have a good attitude and enjoy life. I committed to Exude, to my trainer, the staff and, myself. Somehow Exude gave me back the confidence I had lost. I had willpower, determination and goals—I wanted to look and feel great. I reached those goals, and then some. I looked absolutely fabulous on my wedding day, and most important, I feel great about myself.

The road to success was not easy, but not impossible. Maintenance is ongoing, but Exude made me realize the importance of exercise as a way of life.

MARISSA

Age: 40
Body Type: Cone
Pounds Lost: 30
Inches Lost: 31+
Change in Clothing Size: From a 12 to a 6
Time Elapsed Between Before-and-After
    Measurements: 6 months
Total Time Exercising: 18 months

Workout History: Melissa previously belonged to a health club and worked out regularly. By changing the kind of exercises she was doing and incorporating abdominals, high-rep/low-weight upper-body exercises and the jump rope into her routine, she was able to drastically change her body.

Testimonial: My story begins like millions of others. I have waged an ongoing battle against that extra 5 or 10 pounds most of my life, yo-yoing from an Hourglass shape to dragging around those extra pounds. I could usually camouflage it with the right clothing. A new diet or exercise program would often bring me back to my ideal weight. I can honestly say I've tried them all, some truly ridiculous.

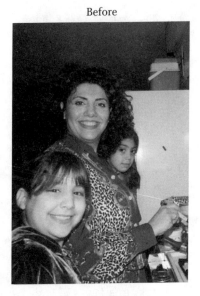

Before

A few years ago, 10 extra pounds became 15, then 20, and then 30. How could this be? I was no longer pleasantly plump. I was overweight. I could not hide my open zippers with a buttoned blazer because I couldn't button my blazers anymore, either. I was tired and puffy looking. My eating binges were not an occasional bag of potato chips, but a bag every night. The weight gain should have come as no surprise. It's what happens when you combine poor eating habits with no exercise.

Every day I told myself I'd start the next. One night on television, I caught the tail end of the "Escape Your Shape" infomercial. I knew this guy, Edward Jackowski. I had worked in the fitness industry and heard his ideas about exercising for your body type. The concept always intrigued me, but I knew little more than that you should choose your program based on your body type. He had a good reputation, so I thought, Why not? I called his New York office to find out more. Turns out I walked by the studio every day. I made an appointment.

Edward did my initial fitness assessment. Within 5 minutes he identified my body type and laid out a weight-loss schedule. That night I jumped rope for the first time in about twenty-five years. My first thought was, This is great! I devised a plan to jump a couple of nights a week and walk on the alternate nights. Walking had been my preferred form of aerobic activity up to that point.

Well, I did a walking workout just once more, because my

Body part	Before	After	Inches Lost
Chest	43	37.5	5.5
Waist	34	30	4
Hips	38	34	4
Thigh	24	21	3*
Knee	18.5	16.5	2*
Calf	14	14	0
Tricep	14	10	4*

* THIS FIGURE REPRESENTS THE INCH LOSS ON ONLY ONE THIGH, KNEE AND ARM.

passion for jumping rope was so immediate. I could almost see my body changing as I jumped. I felt exhilarated like I had never been with any other program. I felt confident. With other programs I was always wondering whether the seat was at the right height or whether I was using the right weight.

I did see immediate results, just as Edward predicted. I modified my diet slightly but sensibly—I didn't eliminate food groups. The best thing for me was that as I got better, I could challenge myself with harder steps. It makes me laugh to hear myself tell others about the program. I'm so enthusiastic about it! The big thrill is hearing the people I've preached to rave about jumping rope and how good they feel just a couple of weeks later.

After

I have maintained my weight loss and I'm confident that what I've adopted is a lifestyle, not an exercise or diet fad. I'm 40 years old and feel better than I ever have. I am fit, healthy and still enjoy a generous diet.

It takes commitment, but I

make the time for me. I feel so much healthier and happier. It's the perfect workout for my busy lifestyle. I enjoy the benefit of a great exercise program and don't spend hours at the gym. As I've already mentioned, I tried many types of exercise and on occasion probably did more harm than good for my body. I recommend you try this program. You'll see results and have a great time getting and staying fit.

NAOMI

Age: 28
Body Type: Slender Hourglass
Pounds Lost: 30+
Inches Lost: 28+
Change in Clothing Size: From a 10 to a 2
Time Elapsed Between Before-and-After
    Measurements: 10 months
Total Time Exercising: 2.5 years

Workout History: Naomi exercised regularly before she came to me for help, but became much leaner, with better toned and defined muscles when she changed the type of exercise that made up her routine.

Testimonial: After I moved to New York from Ireland, I started gaining weight. I went from 130 pounds to 152 pounds. I tried every diet, joined a gym, built a lot of mass, and became depressed about it before—bingo!—I found Exude.

The exercise program they provided has transformed my mind and body in positive ways. I feel healthier, less tired. I've also lost weight and lost inches. My body has changed shape. I went from 152 pounds to 116 pounds; I was a size 10. I'm now a size 2.

My problem areas were my hips, stomach, thighs and arms—basically my whole body! Bit by bit we worked on them and slimmed them all down. Not only did I have to learn how to exercise differently, I had to learn to eat better and healthier. Guess what? Exude helped me with that, too.

Before　　　　　　　　　　　After

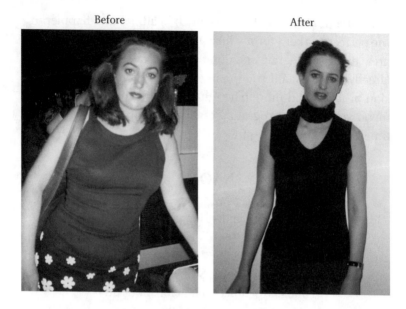

I did have a little relapse after I decided to give up smoking. Exercise became much easier, but I put on a little weight and a few inches. Exude came to the rescue again, adjusting my routine so that I started to lose again. Their staff is wonderful: they care, they work with you, they listen and they motivate you. I work out regularly now and I enjoy it. Who needs a therapist when you've got all that?

Body Part	Before	After	Inches Lost
Chest	37.5	33	4.5
Waist	30	25	5
Hips	38	33	5
Thigh	24	20	4*
Knee	15	14	1*
Calf	13.5	13	.5*
Tricep	11.5	10	1.5*

* THIS FIGURE REPRESENTS THE INCH LOSS ON ONLY ONE THIGH, KNEE AND ARM.

As you read and saw in the preceding testimonials, the Escape Your Shape program produces physical changes, but sometimes the greatest benefits are emotional.

Dear Edward,

While I certainly can thank you for teaching me and motivating me to lose weight, how does one thank a group of people for giving you back your self-esteem, self-worth and self-value? I still well up in tears when I try to find the words to express how I feel after losing 40 pounds. How can I begin to make you understand the importance of what you have done and continue to do in relation to giving people back their lives?

Your staff is all very fit and I do not know if any of them have ever been obese, but I am sure you have had times of feeling "less than" in your lives as well. Now compound that with actually hating yourself for your weakness or with walking by someone who feels like it's their right to tell you how fat you are, or worse, "how pretty you'd be if you only lost weight" and then you know what it is to be us . . . the heavy people who come to you for help.

Escape Your Shape is such a cool concept because the inches that come off make such a huge difference in how clothes fit. When I look at a ruler and see how much 6 inches is, and then realize that I lost 3 inches off each thigh, therefore 6 inches around my body and then 7 more on my hips, 2 more on my calves, 8 more on my waist. . . . Wow! It's overwhelming! It's huge! What I did was huge!

I think part of the anxiety of leaving Exude on that last day was knowing that the program was now mine to continue. I realize it was always in my power to make this change, but we all tend to cede our power to whatever triggers us to eat. The biggest thing you taught me was to put myself first in making the time to exercise, and then not negating all the hard work for a food binge that was nothing short of a self-abusing act. You saw value in me, so I saw value in me. You cared about my physical and emotional state, and cheered every single 1-pound loss with me.

Thank you for being there for me and for all the other people like me who have and will come through your doors.

Susan

The Escape Your Shape program can even produce measurable improvements in people whose medical conditions involve physical constraints, as it did for Jim, who has scoliosis. His mother, Jean, wrote me a letter about the dramatic improvements Jim saw in just a few weeks.

Dear Edward,

I have often remarked to friends, during the past year that Jim has known you and worked with you on your exercise program, that nobody knows more about physical fitness than Edward Jackowski!!! For the past twelve years, since his scoliosis was first diagnosed, Jim had been swimming faithfully four days a week for forty-five minutes to one hour. He did it in order to maintain whatever pulmonary function he had left and to keep himself as fit as possible for his ability. There was never any great improvement seen, but he continued to swim just for maintenance. With three weeks of following your exercise program, members of the Arrowood Sports Center in Purchase, New York, where Jim works out, came up to me and asked if Jim had undergone surgery to improve his back and walking, because he "looks so different" and "he walks better and carries himself better." This is no exaggeration. These people have seen Jimmy at Arrowood for the past seven years.

Jean

Former athletes—who once considered themselves fit—discover physical benefits they could only imagine before starting on the Escape Your Shape program.

Dear Edward,

As a former high school and college athlete, my fitness regime consisted of one thing—running. Strangely enough, I completed two half-marathons in the past year, but was overweight, absurdly lacking in flexibility and had utterly no upper-body strength and poor balance. At age 48, this college philosophy professor owned numerous books on fitness and flexibility, but could not tell the difference between a warm-up and stretching, could not do one push-up and could not jump rope for more than 60 seconds. I dreamed of being fit, but quite frankly, had no clue how to go about achieving it.

Two weeks after we met, I began to see results—I was leaner, my clothes fit better, I saw improvements in balance, flexibility, endurance and self-confidence. I learned what a "full-body workout" meant and I loved exercising consistently with a plan and a set of goals. In fact, with your program, I spent less time working out than I previously spent running, yet I saw dramatic results.

After 4 months we have achieved all of my goals. I say "we" because I could not have achieved my goals without the help of all the wonderful professional people at Exude. I lost more than 17 pounds, toned up my core, strengthened my abdominal muscles, and achieved some measurable upper-body strength for the first time in my life. I am fit enough (I can jump rope for 80 minutes, as you predicted) and lean enough to enjoy running, hiking, tennis and golf with none of the niggling injuries of middle age. My running (while training less than 20 percent of my previous mileage) has improved considerably. Absolutely everything you said about the benefits of your plan (much of which I may have doubted) was true and is true. I feel fit, flexible, lean, strong, more enthusiastic and ready for more challenges. Again, as a former college athlete and sports nut, thanks for helping me get my renewed athleticism back. I truly appreciate it, for you have given me a great gift—the ability to enjoy life at its fullest.

Charles

Midlife clients see improvements in health indicators like cholesterol levels in addition to improved sports performance.

Dear Edward,

*As I have just passed the second anniversary of my being on
your program and have recently had my annual physical, it
seemed like an appropriate time to write and tell you how
pleased I am with Exude.*

*I began as a skeptic, referred by a friend, because I had exer-
cised for a long time and believed that for someone around 50, I
was in good physical condition.*

*How little I knew. Not only has your balanced program given
me strength and endurance that I never would have imagined,
but my cholesterol level has dropped 25 points and my HDL
level has gone from 58 to 74. I have noticed improvement in
several sports, including more agility skiing and the ability to
hit a golf ball farther. In addition, I have lost about ten pounds
and stabilized at a new ideal weight for my frame. All of this in
addition to feeling great.*

Robert

People who have trouble working a regular fitness routine into
their busy work and travel schedules find that the Escape Your
Shape program changes the way they think about fitness.

Dear Edward,

*Two and one half years ago I joined a gym for the first time in
my life. Did I become more fit? Did I lose some weight and tone
up? Did I feel stronger? The answer to all of the above is yes—
with a catch. After a few months the returns on my investment
began to diminish. Even though exercising made me feel healthier, results were at a standstill despite increased intensity and
frequency in the workouts. Classes started to feel routine and I
began to feel like an "aerobics sheep" just following the flock.*

Last spring my work hours changed when I joined the staff

of a news program and worked the graveyard shift. I found the effort involved in just traveling to and from the gym was cutting into already severely limited free time.

When I met you last summer and you outlined Exude's strategy, I was skeptical, to say the least. Your approach seemed too simple to work. For someone to get fit with the most simple equipment (jump ropes and curl bars instead of StairMasters and Nautilus machines??), without even leaving the house, in all honesty sounded like a salesman's rehearsed pitch.

It is now thirteen weeks, twelve pounds and a few dress sizes since I began your program. I find myself working out almost every day primarily because I save a lot of time by not traveling to and from the gym. Being able to go through an intensive workout at home also means that when my job requires a fluctuation in hours, a complete turnover to days, or time on the road, I can alter my workout around the change rather than skip it. I know I put a lot of work into the last couple of months, but it does not humble me in the least to say Exude certainly did the trick.

Judith

For some, the stress-alleviating effects of becoming physically fit are as satisfying as the physical transformations.

Dear Edward,

I have never been so fit in my life! This past summer when I came to you and your staff, I mentioned to you what my goals were: improve my tennis game, increase my flexibility and tone my entire body.

In 3 short months I have won 2 tennis tournaments, but even more impressive than that, have shaped and toned my body in places and in ways I didn't think possible. I used to work out in a gym using Nautilus and free weights. I thought that was what I was "supposed to do." Now I know I was wasting my time and effort.

As a doctor and psychiatrist, I cannot begin to tell you how the program has helped reduce my stress level as well as make me think more clearly. I highly recommend this program to any individual, young and old, to better his or her life on a physical level as well as a mental one.
Barney

Conclusion

To work out properly and consistently week in and week out takes tremendous focus and devotion. Some people have no problem incorporating a sound and proper fitness regimen into their daily lives. For others, it takes much longer. Either life throws an unexpected curve ball that always seems to keep you from looking and feeling your best, or for some, quite simply it isn't important enough. I promise you this, though, if you keep persevering and give 100 percent, with time, you will eventually make *proper* fitness a habit that you can live with. You now know everything you need to know and all the factors that contribute to the success of meeting both your aesthetic and fitness goals. After reading and, more important, implementing all of the advice and information I've shared with you, you are now guaranteed to be on the road to Escape Your Shape. And if for any reason you are still hesitant to follow my advice or believe what I've shared with you thus far, ask yourself this one question: did my current exercise regimen lead to positive and significant improvements to my problem areas on my body and did I look and feel significantly better within thirty days of doing it? If not, your fitness program isn't working and it is not right for you. So instead of pressing on without seeing positive results despite your time invested, try this program. Make a smarter investment of your time and watch your body change for the better.

One final thought. Although I have spent nearly twenty years gathering expertise and the practical experience that has enabled me to write this book, it was *you* who inspired me to write it. You and all my thousands of clients throughout the years asked that I put in layman's terms the answer to your question; "Why hasn't my body responded and does not look that much better despite the fact that I've been exercising for years?" I feel fortunate that you came to me for answers, and I am happy to share with you a proven exercise system that is simple, safe, effective and time efficient.

If you have any questions or comments regarding fitness, nutritional or other lifestyle issues, you can contact us at:

www.exude.com

Or write or visit us at EXUDE Fitness

16 East 52nd Street, third floor
New York, NY 10022
Phone: 800-24-EXUDE or 212-644-9559
Fax: 212-759-4387

Monthly Workout Log

The purpose of this monthly log is to help you organize and track how consistent you are with your core workouts, off-day routines and eating habits. There's also space to record inches and weight loss. When completed, it gives you a "snapshot" of a month's worth of effort. You can easily see why you're getting such great results, or perhaps why you are not reaching your aesthetic and/or weight-loss goals as quickly as you'd like. Before you say something silly like "This program is not working," look at your most recent monthly log and make sure it's not you who's not putting in the effort. Learn from this log and use it to alter and correct your behavior so that *all* of your goals will be realized!

Take a look at the completed sample log on the next page. Below is a key to the letter codes I've used to complete it.

A   Core workout
B   Off-day routine
G   Good diet for the day*
P   Poor diet for day

* PLEASE NOTE: "DIET" REFERS TO THE AMOUNT OF FOOD AND DRINK YOU CONSUME IN RELATION TO THE TOTAL NUMBER OF CALORIES YOU EXPEND FOR THE DAY, NOT TO THE QUALITY OR NUTRITIVE VALUE. IF WEIGHT LOSS IS NOT ONE OF YOUR GOALS, TRACKING YOUR EATING HABITS IS OPTIONAL.

SAMPLE MONTHLY WORKOUT LOG

Date: 10/01/01

Body Type: Hourglass

Weight Loss
from Previous Month: 2 lbs.

Inch Loss
from Previous Month: 4

Diet: G= Good
P=Poor

Total # of Months on EYS: 4

Total Weight Lost: 8 lbs.

Total Inches Lost: 10

Month: October 2001

A= Core Workout   B= Off-Day Routine

Monday	Tuesday	Wednesday	Thursday	Friday	Sat./Sun.
1	2	3	4	5	6
A, G	P	A, P	G	A, G	B, P ——— G 7
8	9	10	11	12	13
P	A, G	P	A, G	B, G	A, G ——— P 14
15	16	17	18	19	20
G	A, G	G	A, G	B, P	B, G ——— B, P 21
22	23	24	25	26	27
A, P	B, G	A, G	B, G	A, P	G ——— G 28
29	30	31			
A, G	P	A, P			

# of Days Diet was Good: 19

# of Days Diet was Poor: 12

Total # of Days Diet
was Good out of Month: 19/31

# of Days Completed Core Workout: 13

# of Days Completed Off-Day Routine: 7

Total # of Days Worked Out: 20/31

The sample log shows this person was very consistent with her core workouts the first week of the month. She did 3 that week. However, she also ate poorly 3 of 7 days that week and performed only 1 off-day routine. At a glance I can see that if her primary goal is to tone (rather than lose weight), then she had a good week. But if she is serious about losing weight, she needs to work on her eating habits *or* increase the number of days she performs an off-day routine to match the number of days she eats poorly. Otherwise, she may lose inches but most likely will not see net weight loss for that particular week.

To create your own log, make copies of a blank log—you'll start a new one every month. In the upper-right hand corner of each box, fill in the calendar dates, then stick it on your fridge or somewhere else you can't ignore. Jot down how you ate and which routine you performed if you did one that day. At the end of the month tally and record the following information:

1. The number of days out of the month that you performed a core workout (total number of *A*s). Here's what the numbers mean: 12 or more = great, 8 to 11 = good, 5 to 7 = needs improvement, 0 to 4 = "it's not working" because you're not working.

2. The number of days out of a month that you performed an off-day routine (total number of *B*s). This one is for those trying to lose weight: 9 to 12 or more = great, 5 to 8 = good, 1 to 4 = needs improvement, 0 = poor and your eating habits better be great.

3. The number of days out of the month that your diet was good (total number of *G*s—for those trying to lose weight). You should strive for good days to be 15+ (fifteen or more) per month when trying to lose weight.

4. The number of days out of the month that your diet was poor (total number of *P*s—again, only for those trying to lose weight). Your total number of poor-diet days (*P*s) should never *exceed* off-day routines (*B*s) if you are trying to lose

weight. You need to balance the additional calories you consume on a poor-diet day with exercise. If your poor-diet days exceed your off-day routines, it will be very difficult to lose weight since your core workout days will be used up to burn those extra calories consumed and you will be only breaking even. Review Chapter 6, "Exercise and Diet, the Dynamic Weight-Loss Duo," which explains in detail the relationship between nutrition, exercise and weight loss.

5. The total number of days you exercised, including both core and off-day routine (As + Bs). If your goal is to just tone, strive for a minimum of 12 days a month. For weight loss, aim for at least sixteen days per month.

Use your monthly logs to analyze and make adjustments to your workout schedule and eating habits. As you progress, you will eventually read your monthly log at a glance, before tallying your month's totals. When you hit a month of great success, focus on repeating that behavior month to month, and you'll be on your way to escaping your shape for the rest of your life!

MONTHLY WORKOUT LOG

Date: _____

Body Type: _____

Diet: G= Good
       P=Poor

Weight Loss
from Previous Month: _____

Inch Loss
from Previous Month: _____

Total # of Months on EYS: _____

Total Weight Lost: _____

Total Inches Lost: _____

Month: _____

A= Core Workout   B= Off-Day Routine

Monday	Tuesday	Wednesday	Thursday	Friday	Sat./Sun.

# of Days Diet was Good:_____

# of Days Diet was Poor:_____

Total # of Days Diet
was Good out of Month:_____

# of Days Completed Core Workout: _____

# of Days Completed Off-Day Routine: ___

Total # of Days Worked Out: _____

MONTHLY WORKOUT LOG

Date: _____

Body Type: _____

Weight Loss
from Previous Month: _____

Inch Loss
from Previous Month: _____

Diet: G= Good
        P=Poor

Total # of Months on EYS: _____

Total Weight Lost: _____

Total Inches Lost: _____

Month: _____

A= Core Workout   B= Off-Day Routine

Monday	Tuesday	Wednesday	Thursday	Friday	Sat./Sun.

# of Days Diet was Good: _____

# of Days Diet was Poor: _____

Total # of Days Diet
was Good out of Month: _____

# of Days Completed Core Workout: _____

# of Days Completed Off-Day Routine: _____

Total # of Days Worked Out: _____

MONTHLY WORKOUT LOG

Date: _____

Body Type: _____

Weight Loss
from Previous Month: _____

Inch Loss
from Previous Month: _____

Diet: G= Good
      P=Poor

Total # of Months on EYS: _____

Total Weight Lost: _____

Total Inches Lost: _____

Month: _____

A= Core Workout   B= Off-Day Routine

Monday	Tuesday	Wednesday	Thursday	Friday	Sat./Sun.

# of Days Diet was Good:_____

# of Days Diet was Poor: _____

Total # of Days Diet
was Good out of Month:_____

# of Days Completed Core Workout: _____

# of Days Completed Off-Day Routine: ___

Total # of Days Worked Out: _____

MONTHLY WORKOUT LOG

Date: _____

Body Type: _____

Weight Loss
from Previous Month: _____

Inch Loss
from Previous Month: _____

Diet: G= Good
      P=Poor

Total # of Months on EYS: _____

Total Weight Lost: _____

Total Inches Lost: _____

Month: _____

A= Core Workout   B= Off-Day Routine

Monday	Tuesday	Wednesday	Thursday	Friday	Sat./Sun.

# of Days Diet was Good: _____

# of Days Diet was Poor: _____

Total # of Days Diet
was Good out of Month: _____

# of Days Completed Core Workout: _____

# of Days Completed Off-Day Routine: ___

Total # of Days Worked Out: _____

MONTHLY WORKOUT LOG

Date: _____

Body Type: _____

Weight Loss
from Previous Month: _____

Inch Loss
from Previous Month: _____

Diet: G= Good
       P=Poor

Total # of Months on EYS: _____

Total Weight Lost: _____

Total Inches Lost: _____

Month: _____

A= Core Workout   B= Off-Day Routine

Monday	Tuesday	Wednesday	Thursday	Friday	Sat./Sun.

# of Days Diet was Good:_____

# of Days Diet was Poor: _____

Total # of Days Diet
was Good out of Month:_____

# of Days Completed Core Workout: _____

# of Days Completed Off-Day Routine: ___

Total # of Days Worked Out: _____

About the Author

In 1985, Edward Jackowski, Ph.D., had a vision for a business that grew out of his love of sports and his exceptional understanding of how to help others become truly fit. With $400 and a dream he was on his way to building Exude (www.exude.com), one of the largest and most successful motivational one-on-one fitness companies in the country.

While health clubs and gyms focus on drawing customers to their clubs with the latest trends and fitness equipment, Edward focuses on giving people what they really desire from working out—results. His medically proven, trademarked and patent-pending fitness regimens based on his four body types are changing the way people exercise forever. Whether you're Hourglass®, Spoon®, Ruler® or Cone® shaped, his gadget-free body-type exercise systems can improve your body within 30 days. Each of the regimens can be performed in any environment—at home, the gym and even while traveling.

As a writer, Edward is a leading fitness author for Simon & Schuster. His first book *Hold It! You're Exercising Wrong* (1995) has more than 100,000 copies in print. In 1998 he was appointed the first-ever fitness advisor and fitness columnist for AARP's *Modern Maturity* and was recently appointed the fitness advisor and fitness columnist for the *New York Daily News* website. A seasoned professional, Edward has written or has lent his expertise to over a thousand lifestyle and fitness-related publications, newspapers, magazines, newsletters, radio and television shows and websites.

In addition to inventing the world's only body-type exercise system, Edward is credited with being the first fitness specialist to educate us on how certain exercises add unwanted bulk to our bodies. He is also recognized in the industry with being one of the first to incorporate jump-rope techniques into a full-body exercise regimen that has helped spark a nationwide growing trend. Edward is also renowned for creating easy-to-follow charts on the correct percentage of aerobic vs. anaerobic exercise necessary to achieve weight loss vs. toning goals. Edward has also invented FastFitness®, a computerized software program that allows individuals from virtually anywhere in the world to exercise based on their lifestyle, medical and orthopedic background, body type, current level of fitness and everyday environment.

In addition his role as founder and CEO of Exude, Edward is the founder and CEO of EYS Productions, which develops fitness products and markets them through direct response, retail and online stores. His "Escape Your Shape" infomercial, which airs in the U.S. and abroad, explains his time-tested body-type methodology.

A generous contributor, Edward donates his time and services to schools, community centers and non-profit organizations. He has also worked with a number of physically challenged children and adults, teaching them how to be more productive by improving their coordination, balance, strength and confidence, enabling them to better tackle their day-to-day activities.

Dr. Jackowski is a much sought-after motivational

speaker. He performs business seminars for companies of all sizes on a variety of business/lifestyle and fitness-related topics. An avid athlete his entire life, Edward also teaches sports-specific mind and body techniques for both amateur and professional athletes, including golfers who are looking to increase swing speed, range-of-motion, flexibility and distance.

Edward holds his B.B.A. from Baruch Business College and a doctorate in behavioral management from International University for Graduate Studies. Edward is a professional member of the American College of Sports Medicine (ACSM) and the International Dance and Exercise Association (IDEA) and is nationally certified by the Aerobics and Fitness Association of America (AFAA) in both Aerobic Conditioning and Personal Training.